Feel Good

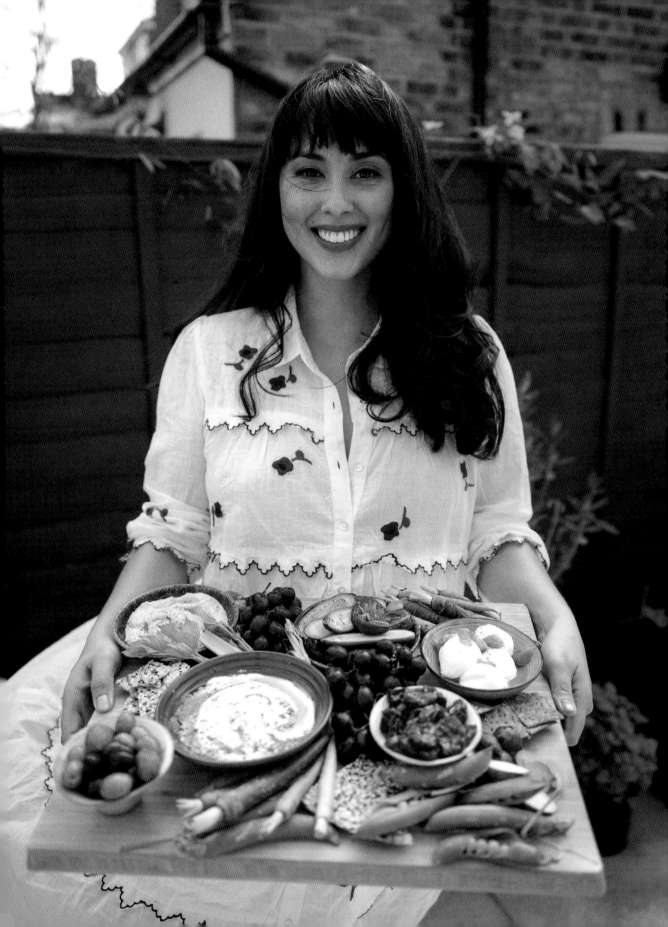

Melissa Hemsley

Feel Good

EBURY
PRESS

Quick and Easy Recipes
for Comfort and Joy

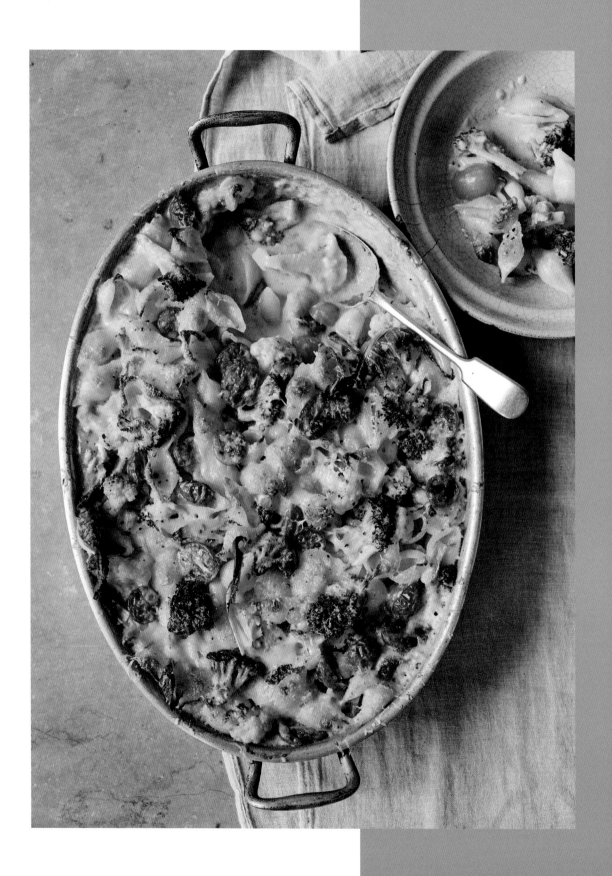

contents

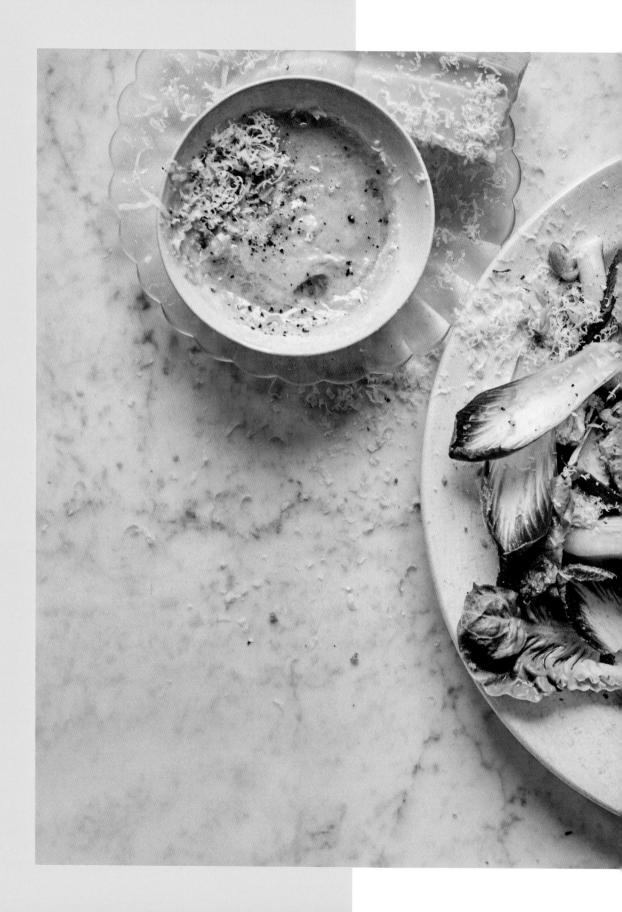

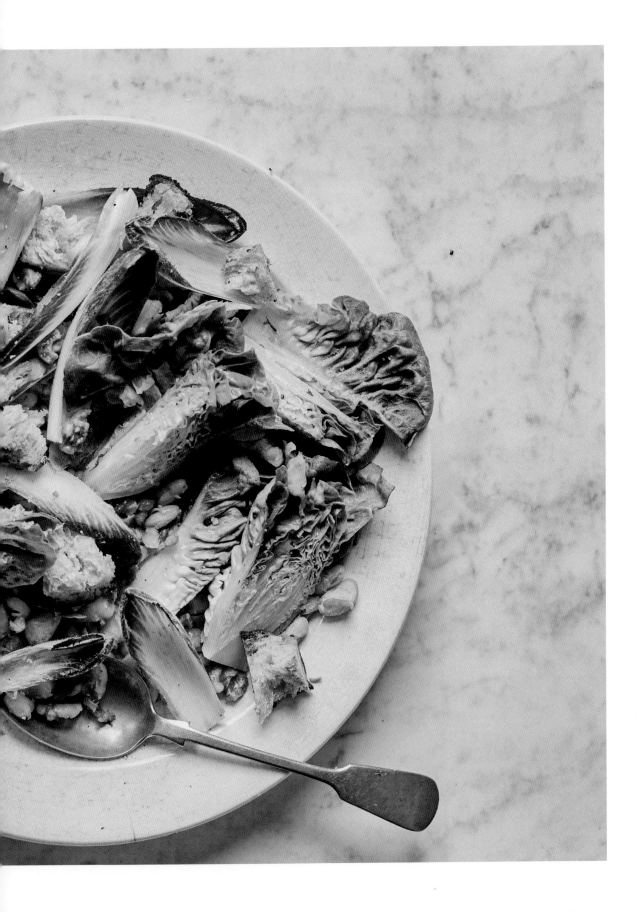

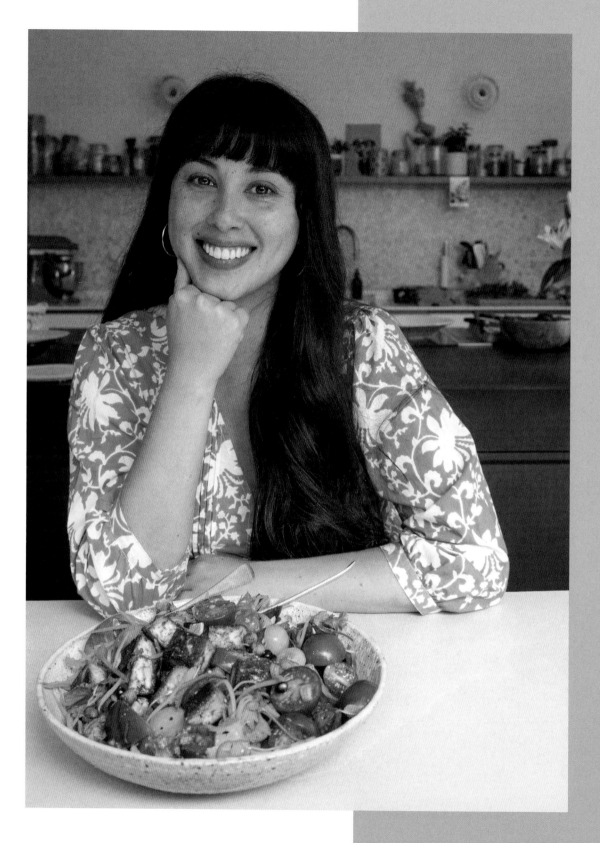

/ the starting place for how I feel has always been my kitchen /

Finding your own unique 'feel-good' is about tuning in to what makes you thrive, and then doing more of it. Feel-good is a vibe! Your mood, your energy, your feelings, your body, your mental health, your experiences, your cravings – you know what sits right with you.

The recipes in this book help me feel that bit better and I hope they will support you too. Our kitchens and dinner tables are great places to connect with ourselves and with others, and mealtimes help us build the positive emotional foundations that power our busy lives and sustain us through the toughest times. Of course, food alone can't solve all our problems but it can play a part in uplifting us, offering nourishment, physically and mentally, and inspiring a little more joy at home.

The starting place for how I feel has always been my kitchen, with something delicious sizzling away and a spoon in my hand

soothing me, even for a moment. It's where I retreat when I'm feeling sad, anxious or overwhelmed (or all three!); it's where I cook for comfort and connection; it's where I potter and prep (as best I can) for those times when I know life is about to get tougher; it's where my mind returns when I'm feeling creative; and it's where I bring people when I want to show love and gratitude, my food providing the warm embrace they (and we) all deserve. Over the past few years, I've noticed lots of us opening up more about such experiences, sharing similar feelings about how we find rest and refuge in our kitchens. Lots of us are cooking with both our mental and physical health in mind.

Feel Good is filled with the sort of easy, comforting food you look forward to at the end of the day. It's a collection of quick and simple recipes that will hopefully brighten up your mealtimes. In this book you'll find reliable recipes that you'll love and can easily make for quick, energy-boosting breakfasts, satisfying lunches and uncomplicated delicious dinners. You'll find a combination of fast dishes, hands-off recipes and one-pan meals, along with get-ahead ideas, freezer-filling options and batch-cooking favourites, all of which can help you achieve more of an ease with everyday cooking.

Feel-good cooking is not just what we eat, it's the mindset around it – a relaxed, flexible approach with no rules. I see it as stepping stones, kicking off with planning what you feel like or what you've been craving that day, then enjoying the process of cooking, however simple and quick it is, savouring the result in all its deliciousness, and the final step, how your food makes you feel afterwards.

While I'm not a nutritionist and nor is this a diet, I like to share delicious recipes with balance and nutrition in mind and at the heart of the plate. You'll see vegetables and whole foods take centre stage. The recipes are all naturally gluten-free (or have gluten-free options), don't rely on refined sugars and there are swaps for those looking to cook without dairy or animal products. Lots of us are increasingly aware of the connection between what we eat and our brain health, so you'll see that reflected in these recipes too, from prioritising a variety of beans and pulses to upping the quantities of leafy greens and oily fish.

As much as possible, I cook flexibly and seasonally and encourage you to give that a go too; it's much easier than you might think. A few tips – don't give up on fruit and veg if they're looking a little tired and neglected, and don't be afraid to swap out ingredients in my recipes if you have an abundance of leftovers to incorporate or 'roll over to tomorrow'. Minimise waste wherever you can – it's better for us, our bank balances and the environment. Plus it's satisfying to create 'something out of nothing' and it feels good to make a positive difference to the planet.

Whatever your cravings, feelings or time constraints – and whatever's in your fridge, shopping basket or energy reserves – I hope you'll reach for this cookbook and find a recipe to suit your mood and satisfy your needs, one that is exactly what you fancy eating for dinner tonight.

/ lots of us are cooking with both our mental and physical health in mind /

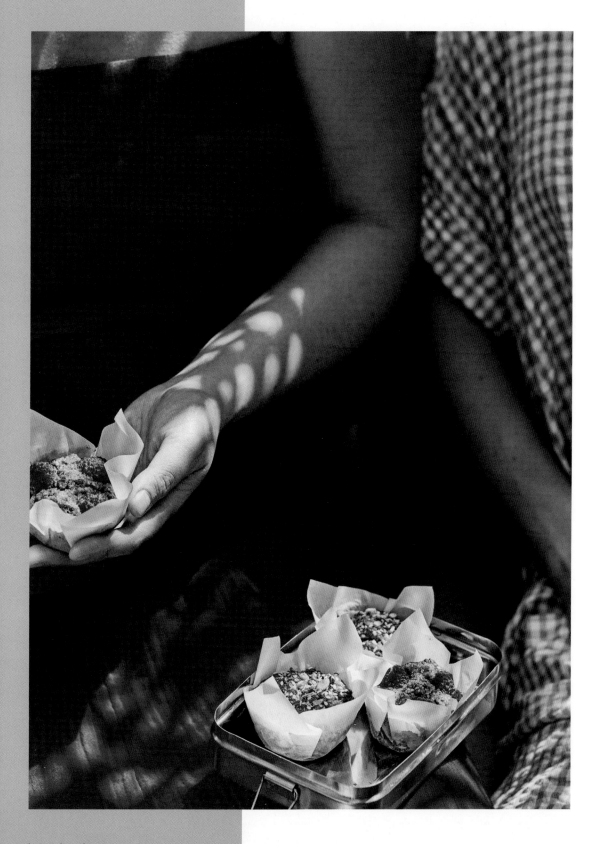

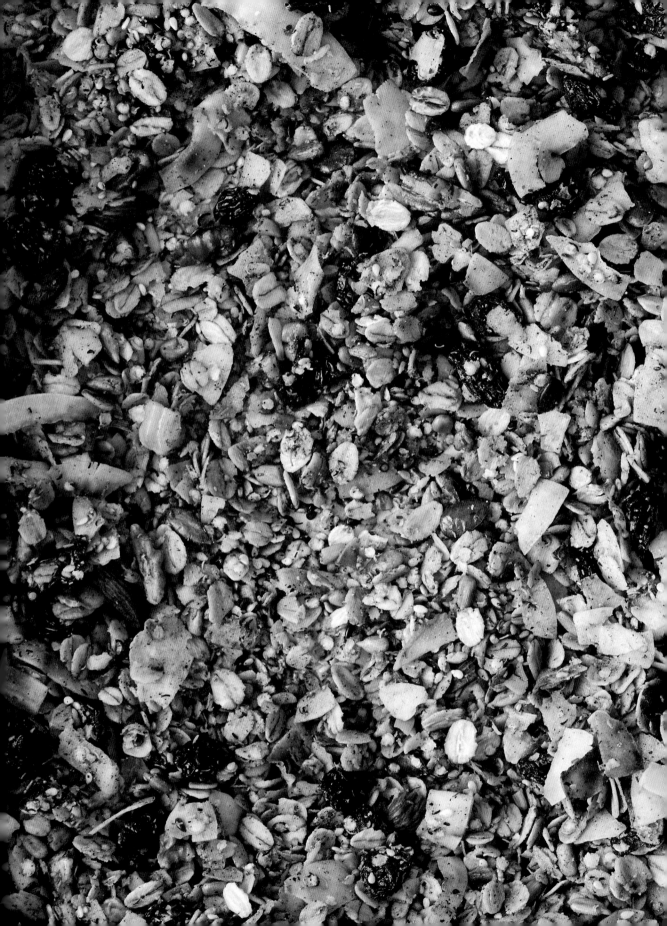

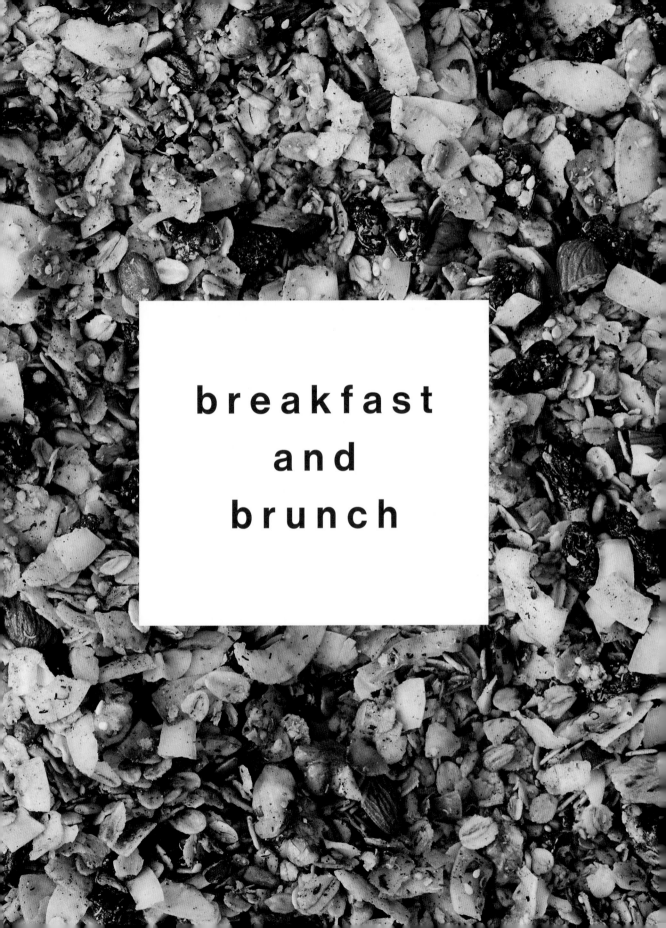

breakfast
and
brunch

/ I'd happily eat breakfast food at any time /

I thought about calling this chapter 'All Day Breakfast' as I'd happily eat breakfast food at any time. Most of these recipes are on the savoury side and if, like me, you're keen to get in as many vegetables as you can, why not kick-start your day with veg! How about boosting breakfast time with **halloumi and asparagus soldiers** dipped into soft-boiled eggs (page 16) or some **Scrambled Spiced Tofu** (a new favourite of mine – page 18), cooked with red peppers and spices? For a grab-and-go option, the **Breakfast Muffins** on page 36 (banana, grated carrot and a good dose of seeds or nuts) keep me energised all morning.

Even though there are a million granola and pancake recipes out there, I couldn't resist sharing these with you – my speedy **15-minute Frying Pan Granola** (page 35), which is gently chai-spiced and makes your kitchen smell irresistible, and the crowd-pleasing American-style **Blueberry Ricotta Pancakes** (page 32). Any pancakes left over can be reheated quickly and easily to carry a bit of Sunday brunch joy into a busy Monday.

And for all those who like a bowl of porridge at the start of the week but get a bit fed up with it by Thursday, be sure to make the **Baked Oats** (pages 28–9) with all the trimmings. It's like porridge but with a bit more going on. For ease, prep several days' worth in advance, changing the flavours to keep things interesting, so all you need to do is to pop it in the oven when that wake-up alarm goes off.

In other chapters, look out for:

- **Banana and Blueberry Bake** (page 233)
- **Quick Leeky Beans** (page 94)

dippy eggs with halloumi and veg soldiers

feeds 2 ———— 10 minutes

4 eggs
150g mix of asparagus,
  ends snapped off, and
  tender-stem broccoli
150g halloumi, patted dry
  and sliced into 8 'soldiers'
2 tsp herb or spice mix
  of your choice
Sea salt and black pepper

'Dippy eggs' are a firm favourite of mine, and are quick and easy to whip up. The 'soldiers' of halloumi, asparagus and tender-stem broccoli accompany the eggs so well and I'm a fan of getting some green veg in the morning. Sprinkle the halloumi or veg with around 2 teaspoons of a herb or spice mix, such as za'atar, dukkah, harissa or ras el hanout. And add buttered-toast soldiers too if you fancy!

Soft-boil the eggs in a large pan of boiling salted water for 4½ minutes on a medium simmer and add the asparagus and broccoli after 1 minute so the veg cooks for 3½ minutes.

Drain the pan, letting the veg sit in a colander, and put the eggs straight into their egg cups.

Immediately heat a large frying pan on a medium–high heat, add the halloumi and fry in the dry pan for 1½ minutes on each side until golden and crispy.

Add the veg to the frying pan for the last 30 seconds to give them a quick warm through, if you like, before dividing everything between two plates to serve.

Enjoy your breakfast straight away while the halloumi is hot. Slice the tops off the eggs, then season the veg and the eggs with a pinch of salt and pepper and a sprinkling of your favourite herb or spice mix.

tip

Save asparagus ends
for veg stock or soup.

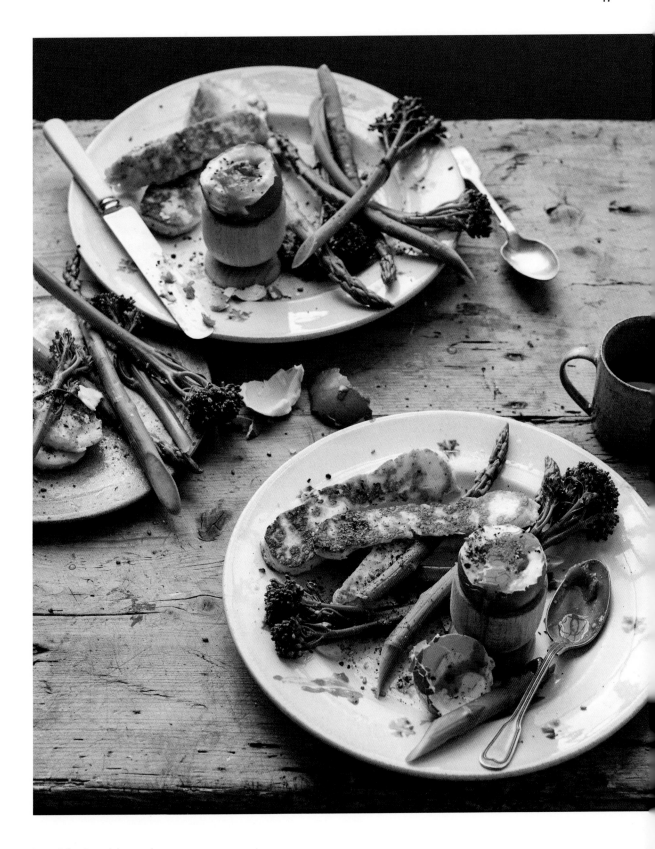

breakfast and brunch

scrambled spiced tofu

feeds 2 ——— 15 minutes

1 tbsp coconut oil or butter
1 medium onion, finely chopped
1 red pepper, deseeded and diced
2 garlic cloves, finely chopped
¼ tsp ground turmeric
½ tsp smoked paprika
A pinch of chilli flakes
280g firm tofu, drained well
  and patted dry
Sea salt and black pepper
1 handful of chopped fresh
  coriander, to serve

If you think you won't enjoy this scrambled tofu . . . just try it! My boyfriend Henry was insistent he wasn't sharing this with me the first time I made it and already had his head in the fridge ready to make his own brunch. Then – ta-da! – he loved it. He couldn't believe the tofu wasn't egg. Add more veggies, if you like: spinach or mushrooms work well. Also fantastic with 2 teaspoons of curry powder instead of the spices. Serve on toast or in a baked sweet potato.

Melt the coconut oil in a large frying pan and fry the onion on a medium heat for 5 minutes, stirring every now and then. Add the red pepper and the garlic and fry another few minutes.

Next, add the spices and season with salt and pepper. Stir-fry for another minute or so, then push everything to one side of the pan, letting that part of the pan sit slightly off the heat.

Roughly crumble the tofu on your chopping board with a fork, then tip it into the empty side of the pan and allow to fry for 1 minute. Stir the tofu into the spiced onion mixture and leave to fry undisturbed for a minute before stirring again. Repeat this a few more times – leaving the mixture to fry undisturbed for a minute before stirring again – to give the tofu a chance to get golden brown in places. After the tofu has had about 5 minutes in the pan, taste for seasoning and add a little more of the spices or more salt and pepper if needed.

Serve hot with the coriander sprinkled on top.

tip

For an extra boost of flavour, add 1 tablespoon of nutritional yeast towards the end of the tofu cooking time or a small handful of grated Cheddar (if you're not cooking for vegans).

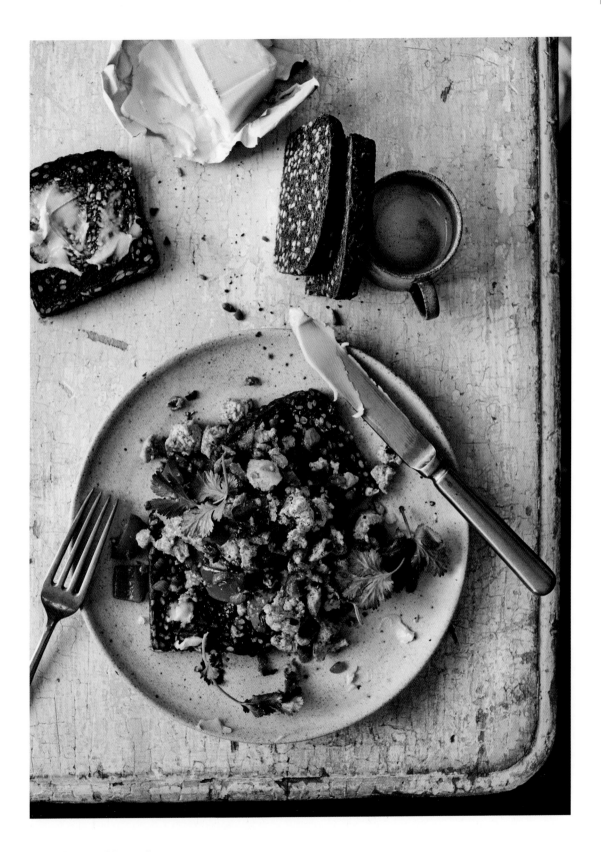

breakfast and brunch

lazy New-York-style eggs

feeds 2 ——— 10 minutes

2 tbsp butter

5 eggs

1 large handful of mixed fresh
  herbs *(such as basil, dill and
  parsley)*, finely chopped,
  plus extra to serve *(optional)*

Sea salt and black pepper

**everything but the
bagel seasoning**

2 tbsp poppy seeds

1 tbsp white sesame seeds

1 tbsp black sesame seeds

1 tbsp garlic granules

1 tbsp onion granules

2 tsp sea salt

¾ tsp black pepper

to serve

2 ripe tomatoes, sliced

¼ red onion, finely chopped

2 lemon wedges

2 generous tbsp cream cheese
  or ricotta

2 tbsp bagel seasoning *(see above)*

When I haven't got the patience for making the perfect omelette or the perfect scrambled eggs, I make these lazy eggs which are somewhere between the two. You could add other ingredients to the egg batter, such as a handful of wild smoked trout or smoked salmon and chopped cooked asparagus spears, fresh watercress or baby spinach. The tasty seasoning is used for the iconic NY-style bagels and is a popular shop-bought mix in America. Make it extra seedy with 2 tablespoons each of toasted pumpkin and sunflower seeds.

First, make the seasoning. Simply add everything together to a small clean jar, pop the lid on, give it a shake and it's ready to use. You can make this in advance, simply shake again before use.

Melt the butter in a medium frying pan on a medium–low heat. Whisk the eggs in a medium bowl with a pinch of salt and pepper. Once the butter is gently foaming, pour in the eggs, tipping the pan to cover the base completely, and then immediately sprinkle over the herbs. Leave to cook undisturbed for 2–3 minutes until just the bottom has set, then use a spatula to fold in half, creating a half moon.

Use the spatula to cut down the middle (this makes the next step easier). Flip each half to allow the other side to brown slightly, then serve straight away, so that the middle is still soft, as it will continue to cook off the heat.

Meanwhile, divide the tomatoes, red onion and lemon wedges between two plates and, as soon as the eggs are cooked, serve up, dolloping on the cream cheese or ricotta and sprinkling over the bagel seasoning and some extra herbs, if you like.

 tip

Try the seasoning sprinkled over avocado on toast or a soft-cheese dip, or with **Farinata** (page 218), **Dippy Eggs with Halloumi and Veg Soldiers** (page 16), **Hummus Bowls** (page 63) and **Loaded Root Veg Wedges** (page 166).

feel good

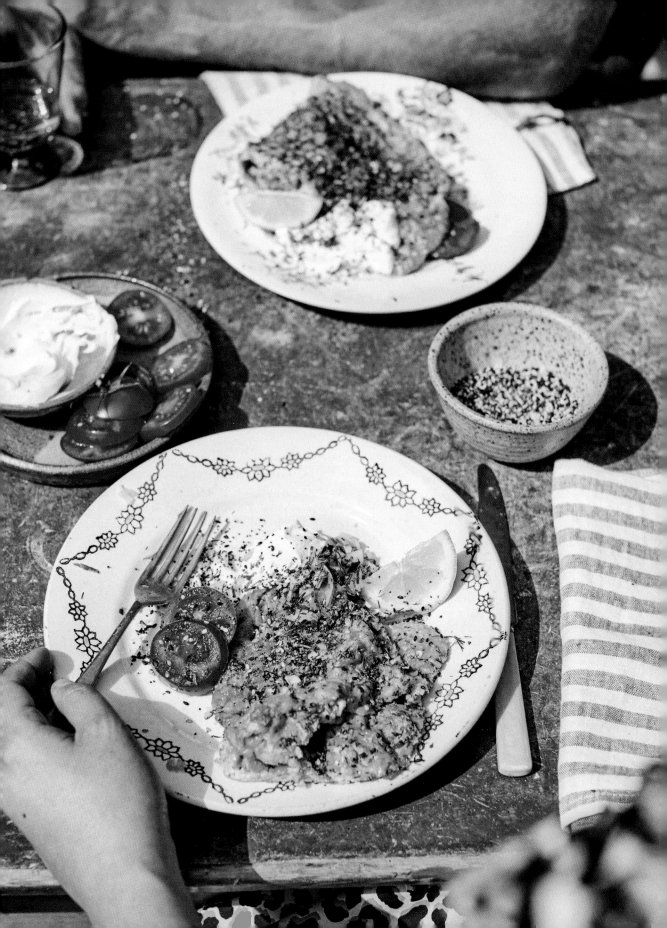

baked eggs with harissa chickpeas and zhoug

feeds 4 ——— 30 minutes

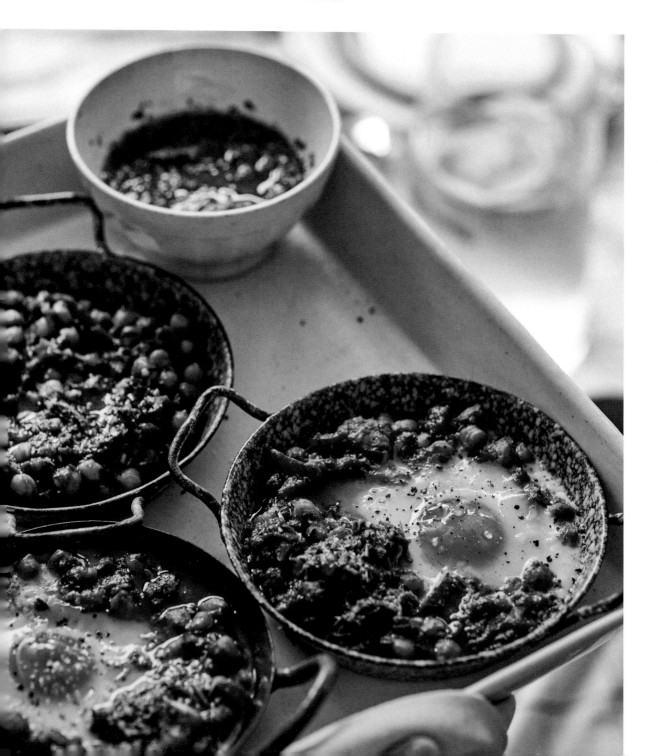

1 tbsp ghee or coconut oil

1 onion, finely chopped

2 medium peppers *(orange and red)*, deseeded and sliced

4 garlic cloves, finely chopped

1 ½ tsp ground cumin

2 tsp–1 tbsp *(rose)* harissa paste

2 × 400g tins of chickpeas, cannellini or mixed beans, drained and rinsed

2 × 400g tins of chopped tomatoes

4+ eggs

Sea salt and black pepper

zhoug

1 garlic clove, roughly chopped

1 fresh green chilli, deseeded if you prefer, and chopped, or a pinch of chilli flakes

1 large handful of fresh coriander

1 tsp ground cumin

½ tsp ground cardamom

8 tbsp extra-virgin olive oil

Juice and grated zest of ½ lemon

A love child of shakshuka and baked beans with a dollop of harissa for a fiery kick. I'd be happy with this for dinner too and extra sauce is wonderful with **veg balls** (page 120). Tasty and satisfying straight up or add some creamy yoghurt or feta. Zhoug, originally from Yemen, is super delicious. This recipe makes extra – it is fantastic on grilled veg and soup too.

Preheat the oven to fan 190°C/gas mark 6½.

Melt the ghee in a large ovenproof frying pan, add the onion, peppers and a good pinch of salt and fry on a medium heat for 6 minutes, stirring every now and then. Stir in the garlic and cumin and fry for another 2 minutes.

Turn up the heat, add 2 teaspoons of the harissa, together with the chickpeas or beans, chopped tomatoes and about 100ml of water (poured into the empty tomato tins first to rinse them out). Bring to the boil and leave to simmer strongly for 12–15 minutes, so the mixture can thicken and reduce, then taste for seasoning, adding a little more harissa for an extra kick, but go easy as a little goes a long way!

Meanwhile, make the zhoug by blitzing all the ingredients until smooth in a food processor and seasoning with salt and pepper to taste. If you don't want to blitz the mixture, finely chop the garlic, chilli and coriander before mixing with the other ingredients.

Divide the chickpea mixture between four individual baking tins or ovenproof dishes, then crack an egg in each. If you prefer to use just one large pan, make gaps in the chickpea mixture (one gap per egg), then crack the eggs in directly. Season with a little salt and pepper, and use a fork to gently swirl the outer ring of egg white into the sauce, steering clear of the yolks. Place in the oven and bake for 4–7 minutes until the whites are set but the yolks are still runny. Alternatively, if using one pan, just pop a lid on the pan and simmer on a low heat for about 5–8 minutes until the whites are set.

As soon as the eggs are ready, serve up, drizzling over some of the zhoug. Serve the rest on the side for everyone to help themselves.

variation

For a plant-based version, use coconut oil instead of ghee and, instead of eggs, break up 200g firm silken tofu into pieces and pop these into gaps in the mixture. Season with salt and pepper and simmer until warm.

baked eggs with sage mushrooms and whipped goat's cheese

feeds 2 ——— 20 minutes

2 tbsp ghee or butter

500g mixed mushrooms,
  roughly sliced

10 large fresh sage leaves or
  1 tsp dried sage

2 garlic cloves, finely chopped

4 eggs

Sea salt and black pepper

whipped goat's cheese

100g soft goat's cheese or feta

100g Greek-style yoghurt

1 garlic clove, finely chopped

to serve

A drizzle of extra-virgin olive oil

A sprinkling of chopped chives

I love this 20-minute recipe at any time of day when I want something tasty fast. Sage and mushrooms go brilliantly together. If friends are coming over, it's worth going half and half with everyday mushrooms like chestnut and wild mushrooms such as chanterelle or shiitake. Serve with toast or the **Farinata** on page 218.

Preheat the oven to fan 190°C/gas mark 6½. In a large, wide ovenproof frying pan, melt 1½ tablespoons of the ghee and add the mushrooms. Fry on a medium-high heat undisturbed for 5 minutes, and then shake the contents of the pan and fry for 3–5 minutes or until the mushrooms have released their liquid and are going lightly golden around the edges. In the last minute, add the sage leaves to the pan. If using dried sage, add now.

Push the mushrooms to one side of the pan and fry the garlic in the remaining ½ tablespoon of ghee for about 30 seconds until the garlic is softened (but not browned), then stir through the mushrooms and season with a good pinch of salt and pepper.

Make four gaps in the mixture (as best as you can) and crack an egg into each gap. Sprinkle some salt and pepper over the eggs and then pop in the oven to bake for 4–7 minutes until the whites have set but the yolks are still runny. Alternatively, just pop a lid on the pan and cook on the hob on a low heat until the whites are set.

Meanwhile, prepare the whipped goat's cheese by blitzing everything together in a food processor. For a chunkier but equally delicious option, use a fork to mash the cheese really well in a bowl, then add the yoghurt and garlic. Season to taste with salt and pepper, drizzle with olive oil and sprinkle with the chives.

When the eggs are cooked, enjoy immediately with the whipped goat's cheese on the side.

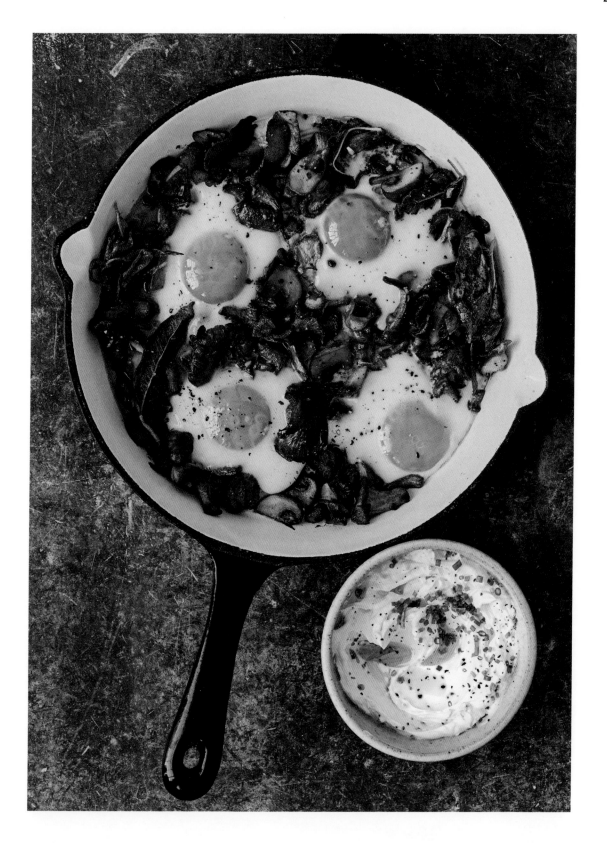

breakfast and brunch

kedgeree-style smoked mackerel

feeds 2 ———— 30 minutes

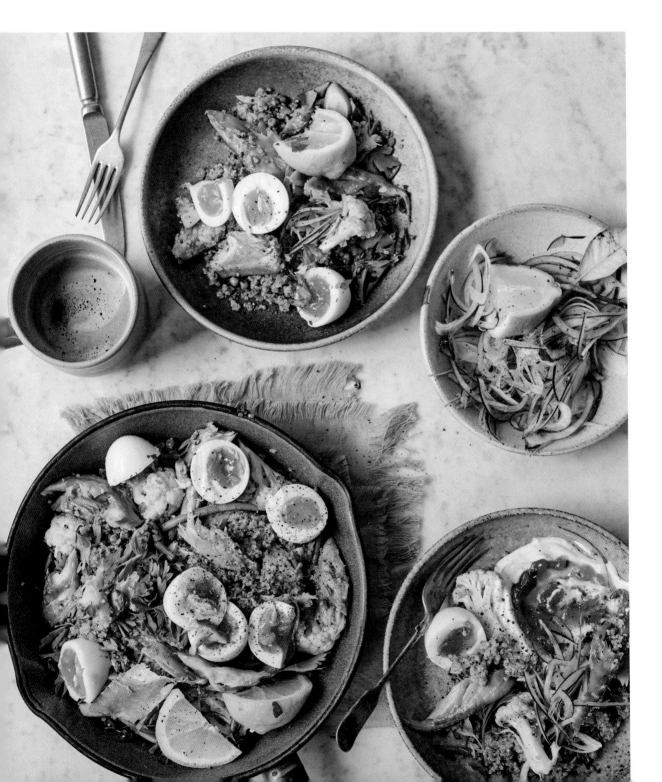

1 tsp black mustard seeds

1 tbsp coconut oil

1 medium onion, finely diced

Stalks from 1 handful of coriander
  or parsley, finely chopped

2 tsp medium curry powder

1 fresh green chilli, deseeded
  and sliced

150g quinoa, rinsed

400ml veg or chicken stock

2 eggs

1 handful of green beans

2 handfuls cauliflower or broccoli
  florets, bite-sized pieces

2 handfuls of frozen peas

2 smoked mackerel fillets

Sea salt and black pepper

to serve

Leaves of 1 handful of fresh
  coriander or parsley, chopped

Lemon wedges

3 tbsp natural yoghurt

2 tsp mango or tamarind chutney

Pickled onion *(page 246 – optional)*

I grew up eating smoked mackerel once a week, and now I see why my busy working mum loved it. The classic kedgeree stars smoked haddock, but I've plumped for ready-to-go smoked mackerel here. Mackerel is generally easy to get hold of – smoked trout is also delicious – and you can add it straight to the cooking pot without doing anything to it first. If you don't eat fish, add four handfuls of cooked lentils instead (a bit similar to the Indian dish that inspired this British version, called *khichdi* or *khichari*). I've used quinoa instead of the traditional rice, though you could also use rice or buckwheat.

In a deep-sided medium frying pan, toast the mustard seeds on a medium–high heat for a minute until starting to pop, then add the coconut oil and, when melted, fry the onion for 8 minutes, stirring from time to time.

Add a little pinch of salt, the chopped coriander or parsley stems, the curry powder and most of the chilli (save some for garnishing). Stir everything together and allow to fry for a minute.

Tip in the quinoa, stirring in the mixture to coat, then pour in the stock, stir, pop a lid on the pan and bring to the boil. Immediately turn down the heat to a medium simmer and cook for 8 minutes.

Meanwhile, place the eggs in a small saucepan of boiling salted water and cook for 8 minutes. Drain, cover with cold water and leave to cool before peeling and slicing each egg in half or into quarters.

Cut the tops off the green beans (no need to cut off the tails), then chop into fifths, add to the pan with the cauliflower or broccoli – don't stir into the quinoa, just scatter evenly and quickly over the top. Put the lid back on the pan and cook for another 5 minutes, raising the heat a little. Finally, once the liquid has been absorbed and the cauliflower is almost tender, add the peas and the smoked mackerel on top of the beans and cauliflower, pop the lid back on and leave for 3 minutes for the fish to heat through, then take the pan off the heat.

Remove the hot smoked mackerel with two forks and roughly flake on your chopping board. I like the skin, but discard it if you wish.

Gently combine the pan contents with the mackerel and most of the coriander or parsley leaves, then plate up. Top with the eggs, season with salt and pepper, sprinkle with the rest of the herbs and finish with a squeeze of lemon. Serve with a generous spoonful of yoghurt, a teaspoon of chutney dolloped on top of the yoghurt and pickled onion, if you like.

baked oats ~ three ways

feeds 1 ——— 30 minutes (*hands-on time 5 minutes*)

These are such a hit with everyone I know! For good reason – the basic recipe is super easy and flexible and, crucially, delicious, comforting and warming. It's customisable, so everyone in your family or your flatmates can DIY their toppings. This recipe is basically baked porridge (with a bit more going on). Use oats or try quinoa flakes or buckwheat flakes. You could also make a few of these in advance and then reheat them; I often do that on busy weeks myself.

I also love adding even more fruit and veg to the basic mix. Any leftover mashed sweet potato, pumpkin, squash or carrot will add sweetness and creaminess to your breakfast. Or grate in apple or pear, add a squeeze of orange juice or some grated citrus zest from a lemon or lime. I also recommend adding a teaspoon of nut butter or tahini or even a little chopped chocolate. In the winter, frozen fruit makes a good addition, and come summer go for it with fresh strawberries, raspberries, cherries, blackberries, peaches, apricots – whatever you fancy!

Each recipe serves one but double or quadruple and serve in a medium oven dish if you like and cook for 35 minutes.

For each of the three options, preheat the oven to fan 180°C/gas mark 6 and grease a small ovenproof dish with a little butter or coconut oil.

Mix all the ingredients (except for the yoghurt) together in a bowl, then transfer to the dish and bake for about 25 minutes or until golden at the edges.

Remove the dish from the oven, dollop with yoghurt and a little extra honey or maple syrup, if you like, and enjoy straight from the dish.

pictured overleaf

1/ cherry bakewell

This would also be fantastic with any berries. I use frozen berries when they're out of season but, when in season, swap for fresh raspberries, strawberries, cherries and blackberries. If you don't have flaked almonds, just chop some regular almonds.

Butter or coconut oil, for greasing
40g rolled oats or quinoa flakes/buckwheat flakes
½ small ripe banana, peeled and mashed
120ml milk *(dairy or plant-based)*
1 tbsp maple syrup or runny honey, plus extra
 to serve *(optional)*
½ tsp vanilla extract
1 tsp ground cinnamon
1 handful of mixed cherries and raspberries
 (fresh or frozen), plus extras to serve
1 small handful of flaked almonds
Greek-style yoghurt or a dairy-free alternative,
 to serve

3/ strawberry chocolate

Any berries taste good in this. I love it with cocoa powder and a few roughly chopped squares of dark chocolate that melt in the oven and add lovely gooey bits.

Butter or coconut oil, for greasing
40g rolled oats or quinoa flakes/buckwheat flakes
½ small ripe banana, peeled and mashed
120ml milk *(dairy or plant-based)*
1 tbsp maple syrup or runny honey, plus extra
 to serve *(optional)*
½ tsp vanilla extract
1 tsp ground cinnamon
1 handful of strawberries or blueberries
 (fresh or frozen), plus extra to serve
1 heaped tbsp cocoa powder
2 tbsp pumpkin or hemp seeds or nuts
Greek-style yoghurt or a dairy-free alternative,
 to serve

2/ carrot cake

Get your spice cupboard involved here for that carrot cake feel or, if you have some chai spice mix, a little would be delicious in place of the carrot cake spices.

Butter or coconut oil, for greasing
40g rolled oats or quinoa flakes/buckwheat flakes
½ small ripe banana, peeled and mashed
120ml milk *(dairy or plant-based)*
1 tbsp maple syrup or runny honey, plus extra
 to serve *(optional)*
1 small carrot, scrubbed and roughly grated
2 tbsp chopped pecans, walnuts or pistachios
2 tbsp raisins or dried fruit
Greek-style yoghurt or a dairy-free alternative,
 to serve

carrot cake spices
1 tsp ground cinnamon
¼ tsp ground ginger, nutmeg or mixed spice
½ tsp vanilla extract
A tiny pinch of sea salt

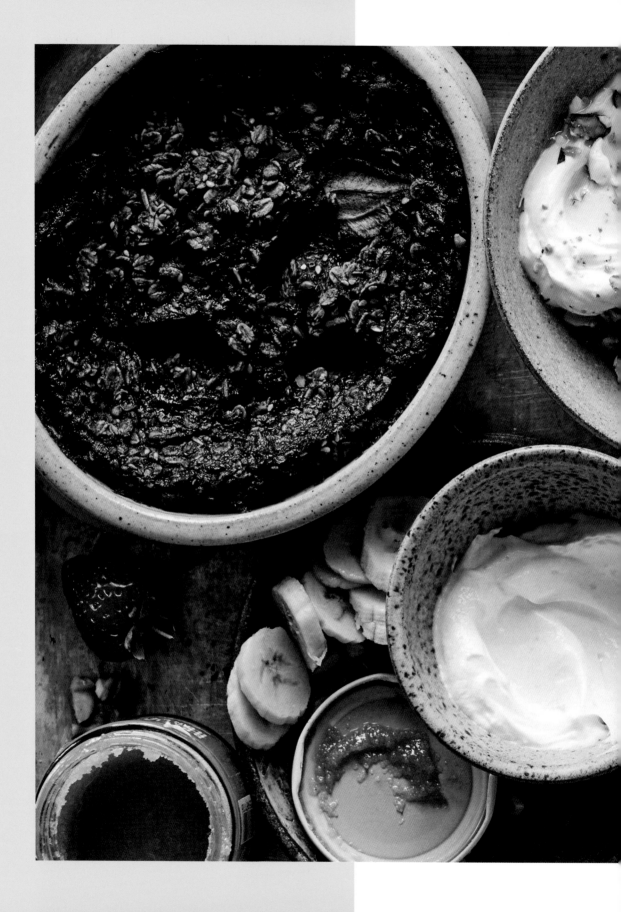

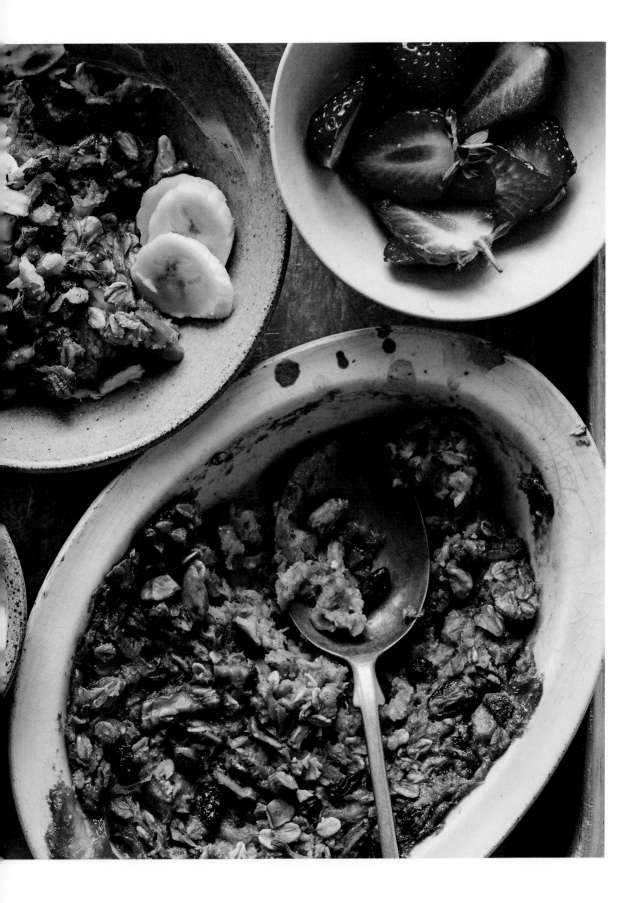

blueberry ricotta pancakes

makes 12 pancakes ———— 20 minutes

3 eggs
150ml milk *(dairy or plant-based)*
100g buckwheat flour
1 tsp baking powder
A tiny pinch of sea salt
250g ricotta
200g blueberries *(fresh or frozen)*
1–2 tbsp coconut oil or butter,
   for frying

to serve
Greek-style yoghurt
Runny honey or maple syrup
Extra blueberries or other fruit
Lemon zest *(optional)*

I love the blueberries in these American-style pancakes, though you could also go half and half with raspberries. No need to defrost frozen berries, if you're using them, which is handy. The batter is unsweetened, so everyone can DIY their toppings. Keep it simple by serving the hot pancakes with cool yoghurt and honey drizzled on top, or with sliced-up bananas or apples and extra berries.

———————————————————

Separate the eggs and place the yolks in a big bowl and the whites in a well-cleaned and dry medium bowl.

Add the milk to the egg yolks in the big bowl, along with the flour, baking powder and salt, and stir to combine. Add the ricotta and blueberries and gently fold in without over-mixing.

Whisk the egg whites, by hand or using a handheld electric whisk, until they form stiff peaks – this takes about 2 minutes by hand. Gently fold the whisked egg whites into the egg-yolk batter without over-mixing.

Pop your biggest frying pan (or get nifty and have two pans on the go for speed) onto a medium heat and melt about 2 teaspoons of coconut oil, making sure to cover the whole pan with the melted fat to prevent the pancakes from sticking.

Add about three or four circles of batter, each consisting of 2 tablespoons of the mixture, at spaced intervals across the pan. Then cook the pancakes on a medium heat for 2 minutes until they lightly bubble and seem ready to turn (resist touching them too soon), then flip them over and cook for another 2 minutes until golden brown on both sides.

Repeat with the rest of the batter – scraping out any bits from the pan between rounds, to prevent them from burning, and adding more coconut oil as needed – and enjoy hot or warm, served with the yoghurt, honey or maple syrup, and extra fruit. Leftover pancakes can be reheated in a pan with the lid on until warmed through.

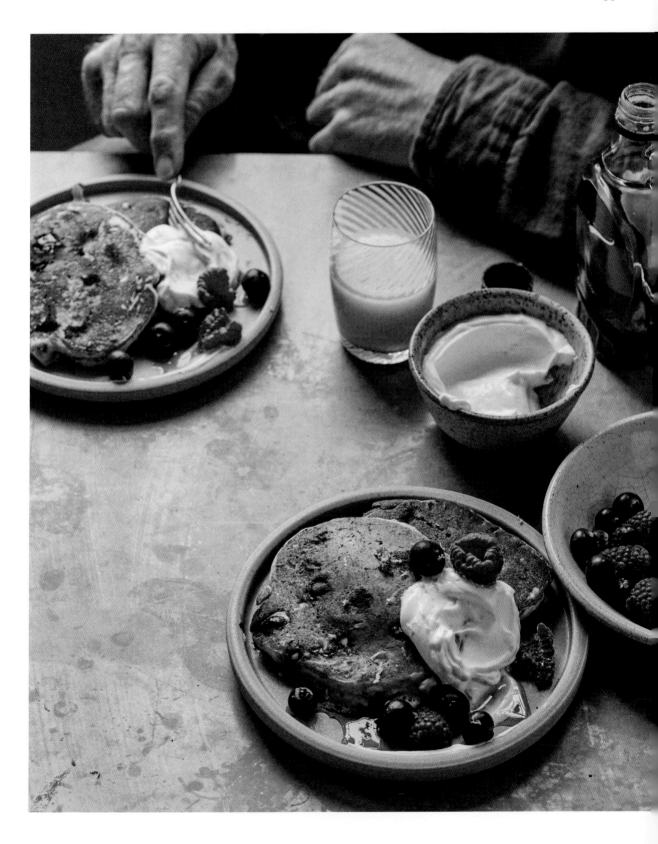

breakfast and brunch

15-minute frying-pan granola

makes 6 portions ——— 15 minutes

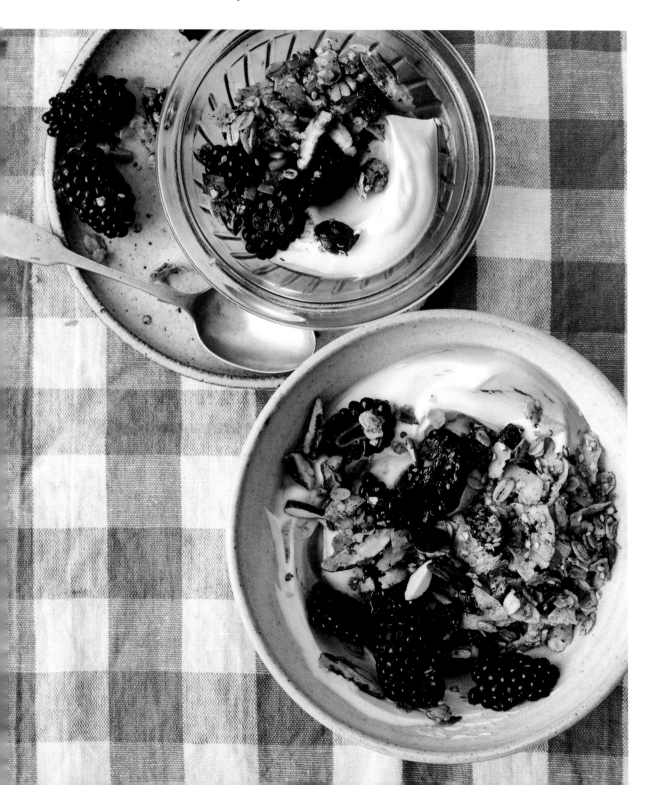

150g mixed dried fruit *(such as raisins, sultanas and cranberries)*

300g rolled oats, quinoa flakes/ buckwheat flakes or a mixture

100g mixed nuts *(such as walnuts, pecans, cashews and almonds)*

100g coconut flakes *(not desiccated coconut)*

200g mixed seeds *(such as sunflower and pumpkin seeds)*

80g unsalted butter or coconut oil

1 tsp vanilla extract

80ml maple syrup

chai-style spices

½ tsp ground turmeric

1 tbsp ground cinnamon

1 tsp ground ginger

½ tsp ground cardamom *(made from the seeds of about 6 pods)*

¼ tsp sea salt

A little pinch of black pepper

¼ tsp ground cloves *(optional)*

to serve

Yoghurt or kefir

Berries

Shredded apple, pear or carrot

This chai-spiced granola is an on-the-hob job, toasting for 15 minutes in a frying pan, meaning no time in a hot oven and more time to enjoy. Use up whatever nuts, seeds and flakes you have and whatever spices you have to hand – you don't need to use all of the ones listed here. If you have a ready-made chai spice mix, you can use about 2 heaped teaspoons of that instead. The grated zest from an orange would make a wonderful addition too.

Put the dried fruit in a large bowl which will fit all the other ingredients as well.

In a large frying pan, toast the oats on a medium heat for 2 minutes. Stir and cook for another 2 minutes or so, until they are golden-tinged and smell toasty, then pour into the bowl.

Put the pan back on the hob, turn up the heat to medium–high and toast the nuts for 3–5 minutes, stirring halfway and making sure they don't burn, then tip onto a chopping board.

Put the pan back on the hob, turn the heat down a touch and toast the coconut flakes for just over a minute, stirring them regularly as they will go golden much faster (watch out!), then add to the bowl.

Next, toast the seeds for 2–3 minutes, or until they start to pop, and add to the bowl. While they are toasting, roughly chop the nuts and pop them into the bowl.

Finally, toast the spices for 1 minute or so until fragrant, then add the butter and stir into the spices as it melts. Add the vanilla and maple syrup, stir again and allow to bubble for 30 seconds before pouring into the bowl and stirring to combine (see tip).

Stir everything together well and taste for seasoning, then leave to cool and transfer to a clean jar with a lid. Enjoy the granola within a fortnight.

tip

At the end of the cooking, I take a big spoonful of extra oats and put them in the pan to soak up any leftover oily spices and add them to the toasted granola in the bowl, so that nothing is wasted!

breakfast muffins with banana, carrot and seeds

makes 12 large muffins ——— 45 minutes *(hands-on time 15 minutes)*

30g unsalted butter, plus extra *(optional)* for greasing

3 medium very ripe bananas *(about 500g)*, peeled

4 eggs

1 large carrot, scrubbed and roughly grated *(about 80g)*

3 tbsp maple syrup

1 tsp vanilla extract

¼ tsp sea salt

1½ tsp ground cinnamon

1 tsp bicarbonate of soda

1 tbsp lemon or orange juice and a little grated zest

200g ground almonds

25g ground flaxseed *(see page 245)*

3 tbsp raisins or chopped dried fruit

3 tbsp seeds or chopped nuts

12 fresh berries *(such as raspberries – optional)*

Very ripe soft bananas work best for these, but if your bananas are just ripe and not soft, then you may need to add another tablespoon of maple syrup. These are breakfast muffins, so are just a touch sweet.

———————————————————————

Preheat the oven to fan 180°C/gas mark 6 and either grease a 12-hole muffin tray with butter or line with paper cases.

Melt the butter in a small saucepan and, as soon as it has melted, take off the heat and allow to cool slightly so it doesn't scramble the eggs.

In a medium bowl, mash the bananas to a pulp with a fork. Push them to one side, then crack the eggs into the empty part of the bowl and whisk well with the fork.

Add the carrot, maple syrup, vanilla, salt, cinnamon, bicarbonate of soda and lemon/orange juice and zest. Mix together with the fork and then add the melted butter.

Add the ground almonds, ground flaxseed, raisins or dried fruit and most of the seeds or nuts, and mix well. Divide the batter between the greased or lined moulds of the muffin tray and scatter over the rest of the seeds or nuts. If using fresh berries, pop them on top now and press in slightly.

Bake in the oven for 30 minutes. If your muffins are getting very browned after 20 minutes, then lower the heat to fan 170°C/gas mark 5. If using fresh berries, these muffins may need 3–5 minutes extra.

Remove the muffins from the oven and leave to cool in the tray for 10–15 minutes before lifting out of the tray and transferring to a wire rack to cool down completely before enjoying.

feel good

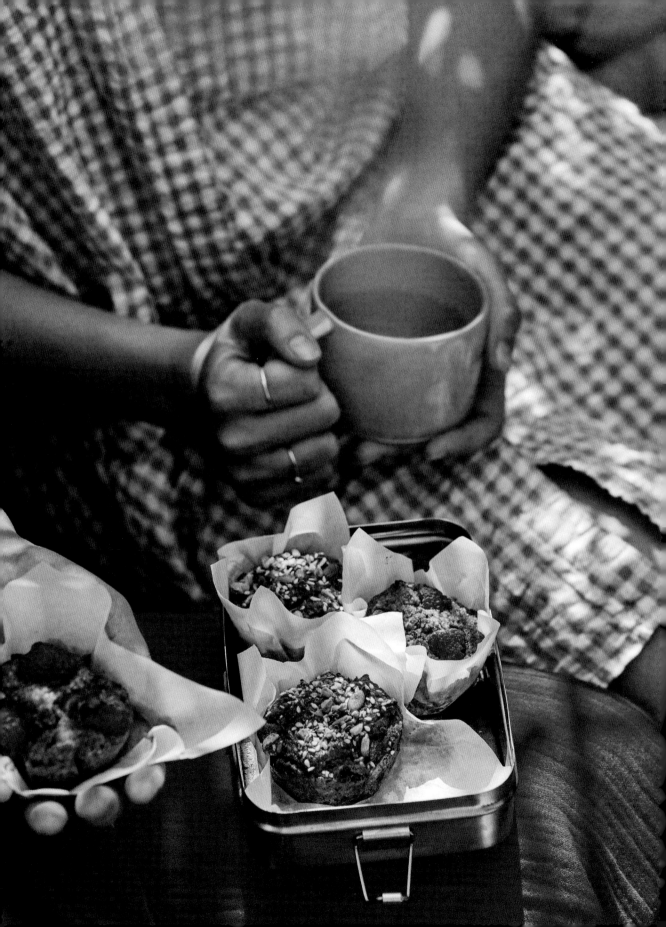

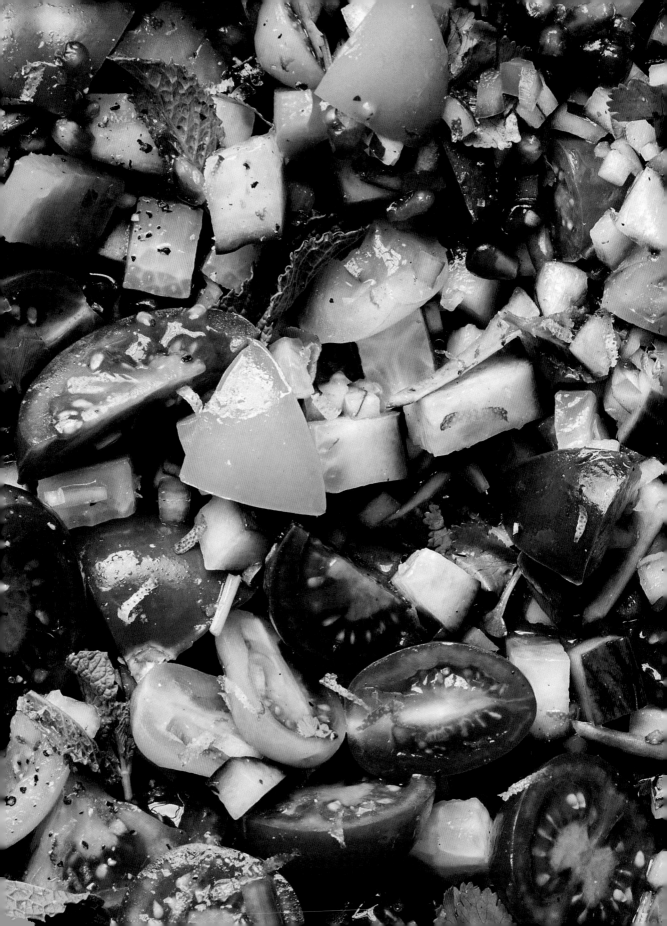

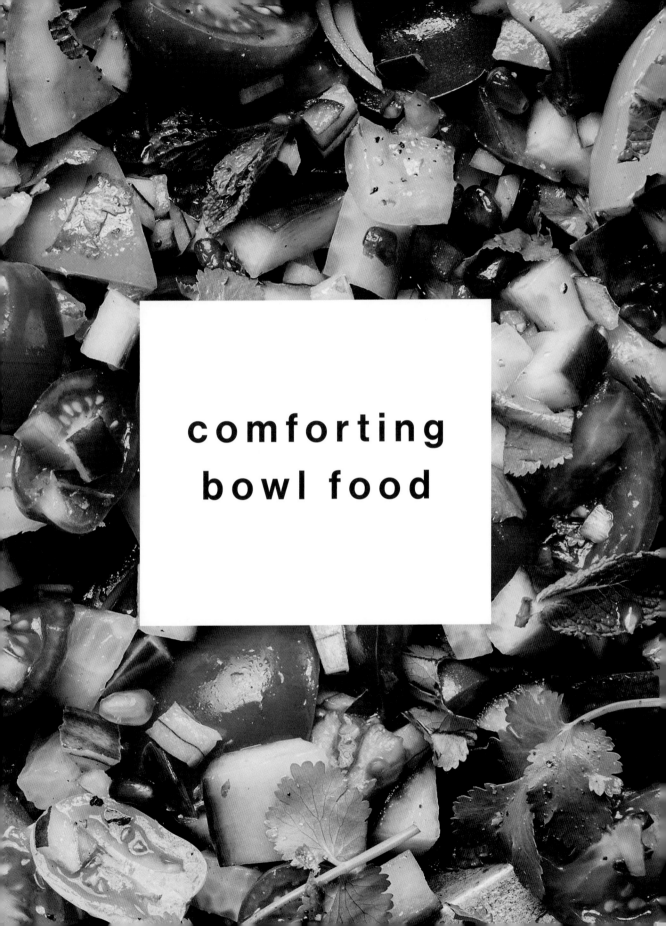

comforting bowl food

/ soups and stews are reliably restorative and nourishing /

Soups and stews are reliably restorative and nourishing, but they need never be the boring or light option – the dishes here are satisfying enough for any meal, any day of the week. In each of these recipes, you'll find a hearty and comforting hot base with plenty of toppings, drizzles and crunchy additions to bring freshness and texture and pack in even more flavour. They're great for some cosy self-soothing after a long day at work, but also special enough to serve to friends. If you wanted to create a simple feast, serve some generously filled bowls alongside a batch of the **Sticky Spiced Nuts and Seeds** (page 215) or the **Farinata** (page 218).

I'm a huge fan of the mantra 'cook once, eat twice', and you'll see that some of the recipes make 4–6 portions so you can save the leftovers. If you'd prefer not to roll yesterday's dinner into tomorrow's lunch, simply halve the quantities in the recipe, or make the recipe in full and then store leftovers in the fridge for a few nights

(where they will get even tastier!), before reheating and perhaps topping with something different (a spicy sauce, herby drizzle, or a swirl of pesto or harissa) or freeze them for a rainy day or a busy week. Your future self will love you for it. An extra portion of homemade food is always welcome in my freezer, and we know just how good it feels to be either the receiver or the giver of a batch of lovingly prepared food. I love sharing food like this.

Don't miss the **Store-cupboard Soup** (pages 44–5), a helpful go-to recipe that turns tins of tomatoes and chickpeas into a family-friendly pot of delicious goodness and which has five different toppings to keep things interesting.

All of these recipes are veg-packed and while I love using homemade chicken stock in my soups, the soups here can easily be made vegetarian by swapping chicken stock for a good-quality veg version – a full-flavoured stock makes all the difference.

hearty spiced veg stew
with toasted almonds

feeds 4 ——————— 40 minutes

1 tbsp ghee, coconut oil or butter
1 large onion, finely diced
4 garlic cloves, finely chopped
1 tsp finely chopped fresh ginger
1 big red pepper, deseeded and
  diced
1 large carrot, scrubbed and cut
  into bite-sized chunks
300g mix of sweet potatoes and
  parsnips, scrubbed and cut
  into bite-sized chunks
400g tin of chopped tomatoes
2 dried apricots or pitted dates,
  chopped, or 2 tbsp raisins
800ml veg or chicken stock
400g tin of chickpeas or beans,
  drained and rinsed
150g green beans, topped (not
  tailed) and cut into quarters
Juice of ½ lemon and 1 tsp
  grated zest
1 handful of pitted green olives,
  roughly chopped
Sea salt and black pepper

spices
1 tsp smoked paprika
1 tsp ground cinnamon
2½ tsp ground cumin
A pinch of chilli flakes

to serve
1 handful of whole or flaked
  almonds
1 handful of mint or
  coriander leaves, or a mix
A drizzle of extra-virgin olive oil

This veg-packed, Moroccan-inspired stew is hearty enough to enjoy on its own, but you could also top it with cooked quinoa, buckwheat or rice or serve with flatbreads. I love it with **Farinata** (page 218). It is also delicious with a chopped cucumber and yoghurt on top. My friend Eva, who tested this, loves the leftovers the next day with fish poached in the sauce.

Toast the almonds in a medium saucepan on a medium heat for about 3 minutes, turning halfway through, until just golden and then set aside. If using whole almonds, roughly chop them.

Put the pan back on the hob, heat the ghee and fry the onion for about 8 minutes until soft, stirring from time to time. Add the spices with the garlic, ginger and a pinch of salt and pepper, and fry for another minute.

Turn up the heat, stir in the red pepper, carrot and sweet potatoes and parsnips and add the tomatoes, dried fruit and stock. Bring to a strong simmer with a lid on the pan and cook for 15 minutes, stirring halfway through.

Once the harder veg (the sweet potatoes and carrots) are almost tender, add the chickpeas/beans, green beans, lemon juice and zest and the olives and simmer on a medium heat for around 12 minutes. Keep the lid off at this point so the sauce can reduce and thicken up, and season with salt and pepper to taste.

Divide between bowls, then scatter over the toasted almonds and herbs and a drizzle of olive oil.

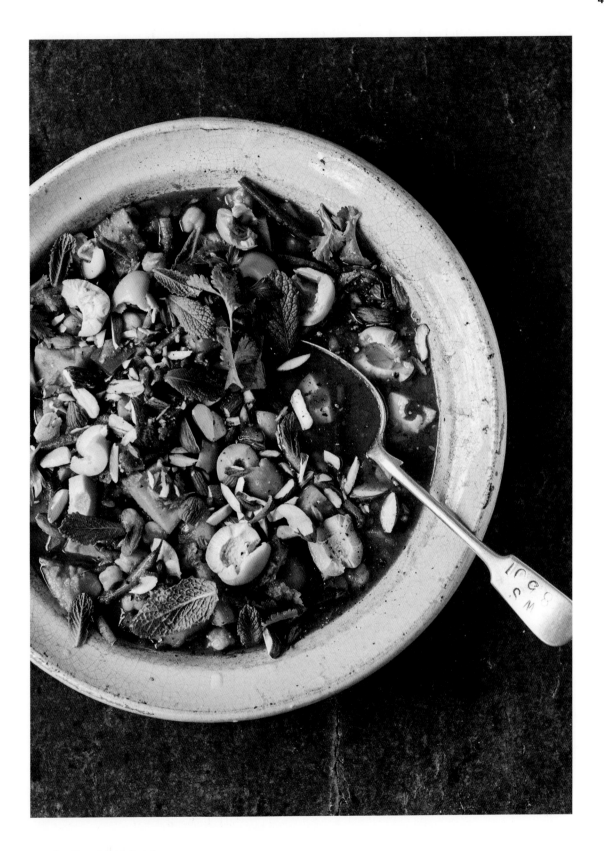

comforting bowl food

store-cupboard soup ~ five ways

feeds 4 ———— 20 minutes

2 tbsp butter, olive oil or ghee
1 onion, finely chopped
3 garlic cloves, finely chopped
½ tsp dried herbs *(such as rosemary, thyme, oregano or mixed Italian herbs)*
A pinch of chilli flakes
2 tbsp tomato purée
2 × 400g tins of chickpeas or other beans, like cannellini, or borlotti, drained and rinsed *(480g)*
400g tin of chopped tomatoes
800ml veg or chicken stock, plus extra if needed
120g dried pasta *(small pasta shapes or spaghetti broken into pieces)*
Sea salt and black pepper

to serve

1 handful of rocket or baby spinach or salad leaves
A drizzle of extra-virgin olive oil
A sprinkling of grated cheese *(Parmesan or Cheddar)*

A comforting, Italian-inspired soup that's loved by everyone. You probably have the ingredients in your cupboard, ready to roll. This tastes even better after a night in the fridge, so why not double the recipe to last a few days, or pop a few portions in the freezer. I've included five topping options to stave off 'leftovers boredom'.

———————————————————————

Melt the butter in a medium pan, add the onion and fry on a medium heat for 6 minutes, stirring from time to time, until softening. Add the garlic, dried herbs, salt, pepper and chilli flakes, stir together and fry for another minute. Stir in the tomato purée and fry for 30 seconds so that it is absorbed into the onion and garlic mix.

Turn up the heat and stir in the chickpeas or beans. Picking out roughly 20 of the chickpeas, smash them with your wooden spoon against the sides of the pan. This will thicken things up nicely.

Add the tinned tomatoes and stock, pop a lid on the pan and bring to the boil, then remove the lid, add the pasta and cook on a medium simmer for about 10 minutes until the pasta is nicely tender (not al dente), seasoning to taste with salt and pepper. Add more stock or hot water if you want it soupier – the pasta will continue to suck up the liquid even off the heat. (If you're going with one of the topping options, make it now.)

Serve each bowl topped with green leaves, a drizzle of olive oil and a sprinkling of grated cheese, and add your chosen topping (if using) to take things to the next level.

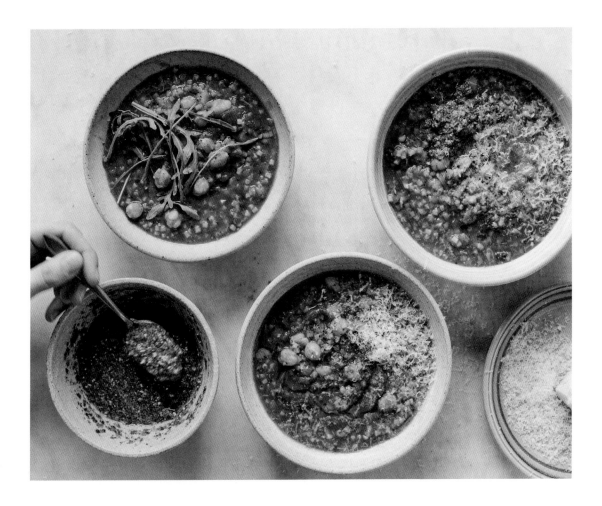

topping options

- **Sage and mushrooms** – Fry 2 handfuls of chopped mushrooms until golden and when the liquid has evaporated, add a chopped garlic clove and 8 chopped sage leaves, season with salt and pepper and top with Parmesan shavings.

- **Herby crunchy drizzle** – Gently fry a sprig of thyme or rosemary, or ½ teaspoon of dried herbs, in 2 tablespoons of oil with a chopped garlic clove, a pinch of chilli flakes and a few chopped nuts, and once fragrant and the garlic is softened, spoon onto each bowl.

- **Swirl of pesto**, shop-bought or homemade (page 123), and some stale bread, cut into cubes, fried and brought back to life as golden croutons.

- **Harissa-spiced seeds** – Toast a handful of sunflower or pumpkin seeds for a few minutes until golden, then stir in 2 teaspoons of harissa paste, remove from the heat and leave to cool in the pan for 10 minutes before scattering over the soup. Add a swirl of yoghurt.

- **Small spoonful of tapenade**, shop-bought or homemade (page 215), or chopped olives or capers, a sprinkling of chopped parsley and grated lemon zest and a swirl of chilli oil.

Tuscan-style pumpkin soup with lemony ricotta and fried sage

feeds 4 ———— 35 minutes

1 ½ tbsp olive oil, ghee or butter

1 medium onion, diced, or 1 big leek, trimmed and chopped

1 celery stick, diced, or 1 handful of diced fennel

3 garlic cloves, finely chopped or sliced

½ tsp dried thyme or oregano

½ tsp dried rosemary

Pinch of chilli flakes

500g pumpkin or squash, peeled, deseeded and chopped into bite-sized pieces

900ml veg or chicken stock

2 × 400g tins of beans *(such as borlotti)*, drained and rinsed

200g cabbage, kale or cavolo nero, finely sliced

Sea salt and black pepper

lemony sage ricotta

2 tsp olive oil, ghee or butter

Around 12 large sage leaves

4 heaped tbsp ricotta

1 tbsp lemon juice and a little grated zest

to serve

A drizzle of extra-virgin olive oil

1 big handful of grated Parmesan *(see my note on using the rind on page 243)*

Sage and squash make a great match, enhanced here by thyme and rosemary. Don't skip the topping – it's extra special. I love the chunkiness of this soup but it's also delicious blitzed smooth and creamy, especially if you're super tired and just want to spoon comforting goodness straight into you. I prefer to not peel veg but it's best to peel the pumpkin or squash here. Save the seeds for toasting and adding to other soups and use veg peel to make stock.

———————————————————————

Start with the topping: heat up the 2 teaspoons of olive oil in a medium saucepan and then fry the whole sage leaves for 30 seconds on each side until golden-edged, then transfer to a corner of your chopping board.

Put the pan back on the heat, add the 1½ tablespoons of olive oil and gently fry the onion and celery on a medium–low heat for 10 minutes, stirring from time to time, while you finish preparing the rest of the veg.

Add the garlic, dried herbs, chilli flakes and some salt and pepper and fry for another minute. Tip in the pumpkin or squash and the stock, pop a lid on the pan and bring to the boil, then immediately turn down to a medium simmer and cook for 12 minutes.

Stir in the beans and the cabbage, kale or cavolo nero, pop the lid back on and simmer for another 5 minutes (adding another splash of water if needed). By now the pumpkin should be tender when you test it with a fork. If not, let it simmer for another few minutes, then take off the heat and season to taste.

While the soup is simmering, mix the ricotta in a bowl with the lemon juice and zest, season with salt and top with the fried sage leaves.

Serve up each bowl of soup, letting everyone help themselves to the ricotta mix, olive oil and grated Parmesan.

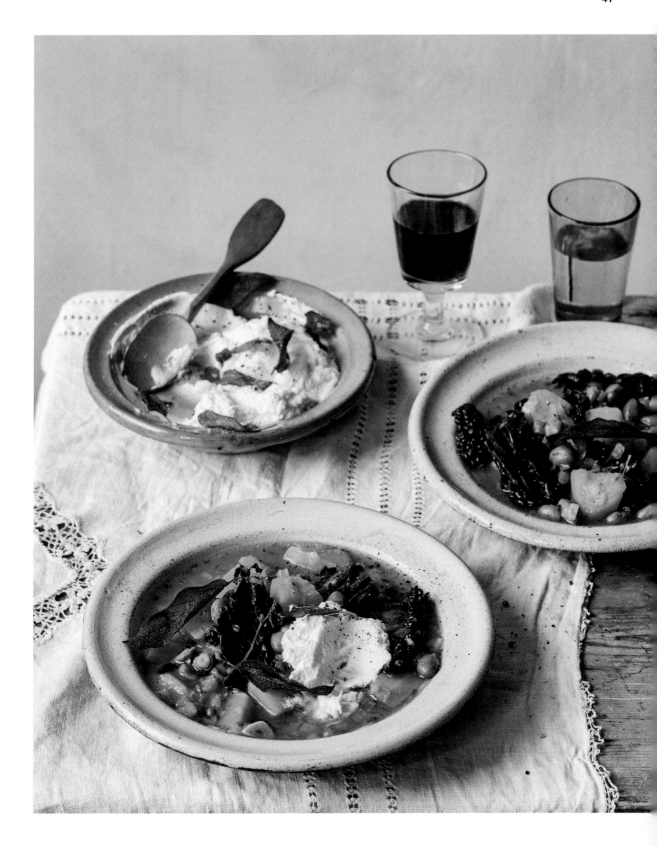

comforting bowl food

cauliflower, potatoes and peas

feeds 2–3 as a main or 4 as a side ———— 30 minutes

400g floury potatoes or sweet
   potatoes, scrubbed and chopped
   into 2.5cm pieces
½ cauliflower *(including the leaves)*
3 tbsp coconut oil or ghee
2 tsp cumin seeds or 1 tbsp
   ground cumin
1 large onion, finely chopped
4 big garlic cloves, finely chopped
2.5cm fresh ginger, finely grated
2 tsp ground coriander
½ tsp ground turmeric
1 tsp garam masala
1 fresh green chilli, deseeded
   and sliced
400g tin of chopped tomatoes
2 handfuls of coriander, stalks
   finely chopped and leaves whole
2 handfuls of frozen peas
Sea salt

optional extras
Lime wedges
Natural yoghurt
Chutney *(such as the Freestyle
   Fruit-Bowl Chutney on page 247)*

Loosely inspired by *aloo gobi*, I've added the cauliflower leaves too (no waste) and frozen peas for extra greens and a little sweetness. This recipe uses potatoes but I'll sometimes swap them for sweet potatoes, depending on what needs using up. You can serve this as a side, though I love a big bowl of it on its own. Leftovers are fantastic in a wrap or with a fried egg and a dollop of **chutney** (page 247).

———————————————————————

Bring a medium saucepan of well-salted water to the boil. Carefully drop the potatoes or sweet potatoes into the boiling water and cook until just tender. Potatoes take 12–15 minutes and sweet potatoes slightly less time. Drain in a colander and set aside.

Meanwhile, prepare the cauliflower by chopping into bite-sized florets and finely slicing the stem and leaves. Heat up the coconut oil in a large, deep-sided frying pan and fry the cumin seeds, if using, for 10 seconds before adding the onion and a pinch of salt, then fry on a medium heat, stirring every now and then, for 5 minutes until beginning to soften. Add the cauliflower florets and stems (not the leaves) and fry for 10 minutes, stirring every now and then.

Add the garlic and ginger and fry for a minute, then add the spices including the ground cumin, if using, and chilli and stir well.

Stir in the finely chopped cauliflower leaves (about 1 big handful), the tinned tomatoes and the coriander stalks, then turn up the heat and let the mixture bubble away strongly for 5 minutes. If it looks dry, add some water to the tomato tin, give it a swirl and add it to the pan.

Add the boiled potatoes and allow to cook for 5 minutes until the sauce has reduced and the vegetables are tender but still holding their shape. Taste for seasoning and check that the veg are tender – if they need a little longer, add a splash of water and continue to cook for another couple of minutes. Stir in the frozen peas and allow to cook for a minute until thawed and hot, then take the pan off the heat. Serve with the coriander leaves and any of the optional extras.

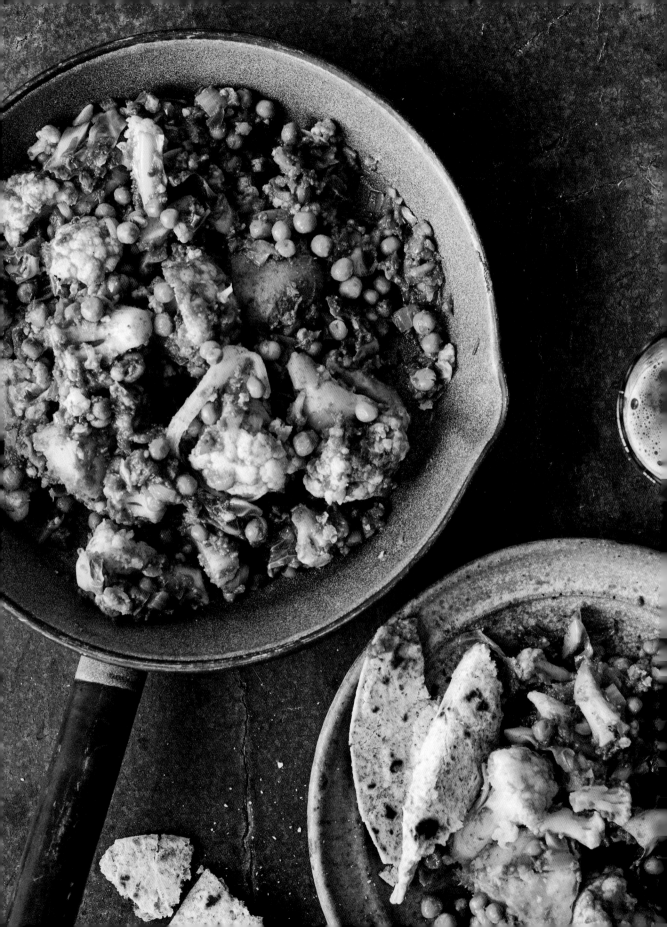

spring vegetable noodle broth with miso-ginger drizzle

feeds 2 ——— 25 minutes

2 garlic cloves, finely sliced
2 tsp finely grated fresh ginger
4 spring onions, thinly sliced
2 tsp coconut oil
120g shiitake mushrooms,
  roughly sliced
800ml veg or chicken stock
2 big handfuls of asparagus,
  green beans or broccoli
100g baby spinach, finely sliced
2 bundles of dried soba noodles
Sea salt

miso-ginger drizzle

3 tbsp apple cider vinegar
1½ tbsp white miso paste *(to taste)*
2 tbsp black sesame seeds
2 tsp finely grated fresh ginger
A pinch of chilli flakes or finely
  chopped fresh chilli

to serve

1 tbsp tamari or soy sauce *(to taste)*
1 handful of radishes, thinly sliced
4 ribbons of cucumber *(made
  using a vegetable peeler)*
2 soft-boiled eggs *(cooked for about
  7 minutes)*, halved

variation

For a winter version, use leeks, cauliflower florets and cavolo nero or other dark leafy greens. Simmer for about 8 minutes until just tender.

Full-flavoured restorative noodle soup in a flash. The miso-ginger drizzle is tangy, salty and just sweet enough from the white miso. You'll be wanting to drizzle it over everything; it really livens up leftovers. Soba noodles (Japanese buckwheat noodles) are amazing in this, but use any noodles you like.

Mix the ingredients for the miso-ginger drizzle together in a small bowl. Add a little pinch of sea salt and set aside.

In a medium saucepan, gently fry the garlic, ginger and sliced spring onions (saving a few spring onion slices to serve) in the coconut oil for 2 minutes, stirring occasionally. Add the mushrooms and a little sea salt and stir-fry for 2 minutes.

Add the stock and cover with a lid, then turn up the heat and bring to a medium simmer. Cook for about 5 minutes, then take off the lid, add the green vegetables and cook for 3–4 minutes until the veg are bright green and just tender, then remove from the heat.

Meanwhile, bring a saucepan of water to the boil, add the noodles and cook in strongly simmering water for around 5 minutes (or according to the packet instructions). I normally undercook them by a minute as they will cook more when added to the soup.

Ladle the soup into big bowls, then add the noodles, swirl in the miso-ginger drizzle and taste for seasoning. If you'd like an extra salty, umami flavour hit, add 1 or 2 teaspoons of tamari or soy sauce. Top with the sliced radish, cucumber ribbons, halved soft-boiled egg and reserved spring onion slices.

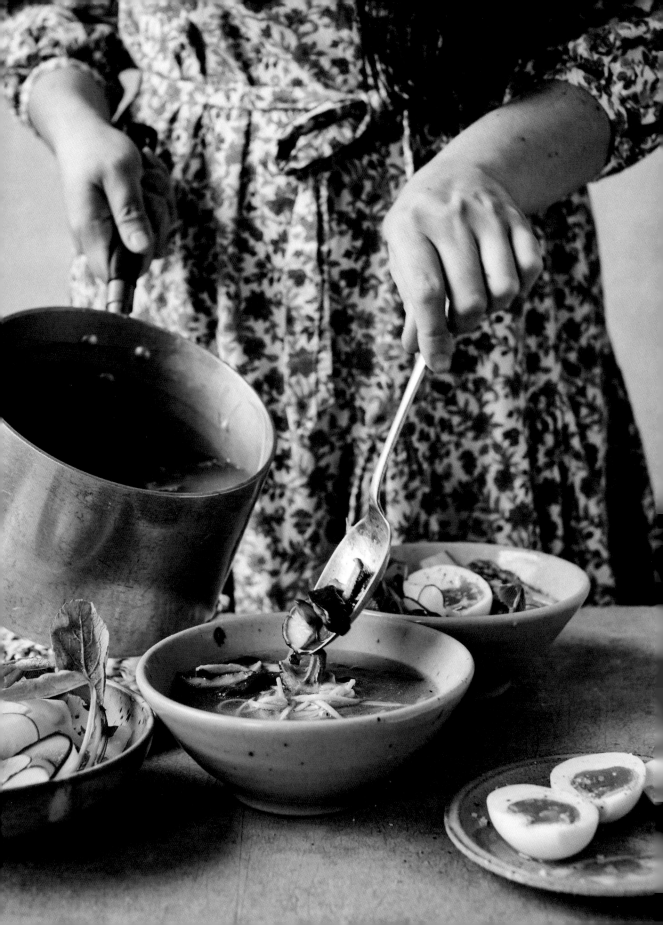

broccoli coconut curry soup

feeds 4 ———— 30 minutes

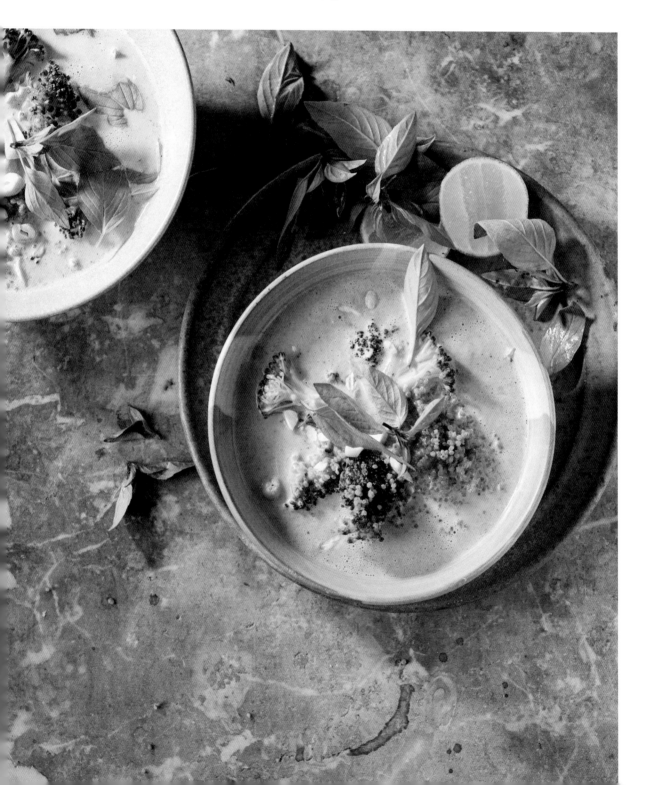

1 handful of cashews

2 tbsp coconut oil or ghee

1 tsp ground cumin

½ tsp ground turmeric

2 tsp fish sauce *(vegan if you prefer)*

400ml tin of coconut milk

1 large head of broccoli

Juice of 1 lime

Sea salt and black pepper

green curry paste

1 large onion or 3 shallots

4 garlic cloves, peeled

2 lemongrass stalks, outer leaves
  discarded

1–2 fresh green chillies *(to taste)*,
  deseeded if you prefer

5cm fresh ginger

2 large handfuls of fresh coriander,
  stalks and leaves separated

Grated zest of 1 lime

optional extras

4 lime wedges

Fresh herbs *(such as Thai basil)*

4 big spoonfuls of cooked quinoa
  or rice

Inspired by Thai green curry, this is a delicious soup that can be topped with cooked buckwheat, quinoa, chickpeas or noodles. Broccoli is the star here, but any other veg could be included too, such as sweetcorn, asparagus or baby spinach – simply add them with the broccoli. You can also make it heartier with fried mushrooms, roasted tofu, fish or leftover shredded chicken.

Heat up a frying pan and toast the cashews on a medium heat for a few minutes until golden.

Roughly chop all the ingredients for the paste except the lime, chopping them more finely if you know your food processor may need a bit of help. Add everything to the food processor except for the coriander leaves and go easy on the fresh chilli as you can always add more if needed. Blitz until broken down into a paste, adding a tablespoon of water if it needs loosening a little.

Melt the coconut oil in a large saucepan, stir in the paste – a spatula helps here to get everything out of the food processor – and stir-fry on a medium heat for 3–4 minutes until fragrant.

Add the spices and a good pinch of salt and pepper, and stir-fry for a minute. Add the fish sauce and coconut milk, then fill the empty coconut milk tin with water (400ml) and pour that in too. Stir it all together well, turn up the heat, pop a lid on the pan and bring to a medium simmer to cook for 10 minutes.

Chop the broccoli into even-sized florets and finely slice the stalk. After the mixture in the pan has been simmering for 10 minutes, remove the lid, add the broccoli stems and florets (as well as any other veg – see introduction) and simmer for 6 minutes until the broccoli stems are tender to the point of a knife.

Take the pan off the heat, add the lime juice and taste for seasoning (see tip). Divide the soup between bowls, top with the toasted cashews and add the optional extras, if using.

tip

I really recommend making this simple curry paste, but if you're in a rush, swap it for 2 tablespoons of shop-bought green curry paste, checking the label as some brands are spicier and saltier than others.

comforting bowl food

beans and greens golden broth

feeds 4 heartily ——— 35 minutes

2 tbsp ghee, butter or olive oil
1 onion or leek, finely chopped
4cm fresh ginger, finely chopped
4 garlic cloves, finely chopped
1 tsp ground turmeric
1 tsp ground coriander
Seeds from 2 cardamom pods
1 star anise or ½ tsp Chinese
   five-spice powder
A pinch of chilli flakes
500g mix of carrots and potatoes
   or sweet potatoes, scrubbed and
   diced into 1cm pieces
1.3 litres veg or chicken stock
2 × 400g tins of mixed beans
   (such as cannellini and haricot),
   drained and rinsed
200g kale or cavolo nero leaves,
   finely shredded
Juice of ⅓ lemon or ½ lime
Sea salt and black pepper

zesty salted yoghurt
Natural or coconut yoghurt
A little grated lemon or lime zest

A beautifully-spiced and hearty one-pot dish of brothy beans with lots of greens. Use fresh kale and save the stems for another recipe, such as **Pesto** (page 123) or a stir-fry; otherwise I use frozen kale, which makes this recipe an excellent store-cupboard and freezer staple. In the summer, I swap the kale for baby spinach and add spring onions and fresh herbs such as chives. I recommend you use a full-flavoured vegetable or chicken stock, as good soups need a good base!

———————————————————————

Heat up a medium saucepan, add the ghee and fry the onion or leek on a medium heat for about 8 minutes, stirring regularly.

Add the ginger, garlic, spices, chilli flakes, salt and pepper and stir-fry for a minute. Add the carrots and potatoes or sweet potatoes, pour in the stock, put a lid on the pan and bring to a strong simmer to cook for 15 minutes, stirring halfway through.

Tip in the beans, give the pan a stir, then put the lid back on and simmer for 5 minutes. Add the kale or cavolo nero and simmer for another 5 minutes until tender. Add the lemon or lime juice and season with salt and pepper to taste.

Serve up each bowl with a spoonful of yoghurt topped with the citrus zest and a light sprinkling of salt.

tip

I like how brothy this is, but if you prefer it less slurpy, use less stock or blitz the soup with a handheld blender, or just blitz a few ladlefuls of the soup and then pour it back into the pan.

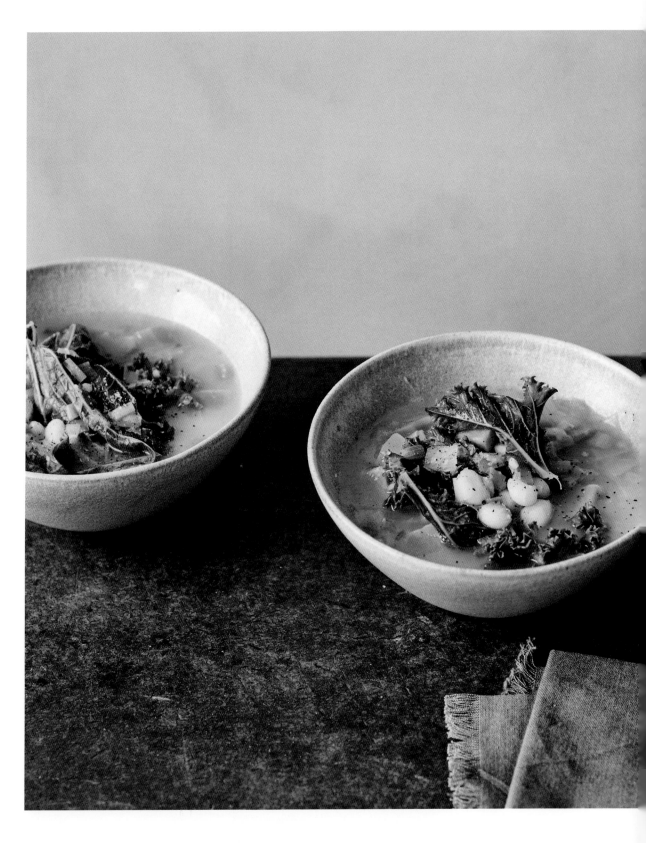

comforting bowl food

fried-up quinoa leftovers bowl

feeds 2 ——— 20 minutes

1 ½ tbsp coconut oil

1 shallot or ½ red onion, sliced

2 garlic cloves, finely chopped

2cm fresh ginger, finely grated
   or chopped

1 small head of broccoli

1 handful of green beans or
   shredded cabbage

3 spring onions

A pinch of chilli flakes or a little
   chopped fresh chilli

¼ tsp ground turmeric

250g cooked quinoa or rice

2 tsp fish sauce *(vegan if you prefer)*

2 tbsp kecap manis *(or 1 ½ tbsp
   tamari or soy sauce + 2 tsp
   maple syrup)*

2 eggs

Sea salt and black pepper

to serve

2 tbsp peanuts or cashews

Sliced cucumber

2 lime wedges

This came about from craving fried rice one evening but finding I had no leftover rice, so quinoa came to the rescue! It is inspired by *nasi goreng*, the delicious Indonesian dish, and makes an excellent vehicle for all sorts of veg. If you don't have leftover rice or quinoa, cook up 100g and let it cool completely before putting it in the fridge to chill for a few hours. This is delicious with **Omelette Ribbons** (page 132).

Heat up a large frying pan or wok and toast the peanuts or cashews on a medium heat for a few minutes until golden, then set aside.

Put the pan back on the heat with 1 tablespoon of the coconut oil, add the shallot or red onion, garlic and ginger and stir-fry on a medium–high heat for 3 minutes.

Meanwhile, prepare the veg. Chop the broccoli into bite-sized florets and finely slice the stem pieces. Top (but don't tail) the green beans, if using, and chop them into thirds, then slice the spring onions. Add the veg to the pan, keeping back some of the spring onions for garnishing, along with the chilli and turmeric, and stir-fry for a few minutes.

Turn the heat right up and tip the quinoa (or rice) into the pan, breaking it up with your hands or with a spoon as you add it. Mix everything together and then stir-fry on a high heat for 3 minutes; if you end up with a few golden-edged bits of quinoa, then even better. Drizzle in the fish sauce and kecap manis and taste for seasoning – you might want to add salt or a little more kecap manis.

Once the veg are tender, divide everything between two bowls, scraping out and adding the delicious bits on the bottom of the pan.

Put the pan straight back onto the heat and melt the remaining ½ tablespoon of coconut oil. Once the oil is hot, crack in the eggs, season with a little salt, and fry them on a medium-high heat until crispy-edged, then season with salt and pepper and slide the eggs onto your fried quinoa. Serve with the toasted nuts, roughly chopped, and some sliced cucumber and with the rest of the spring onions scattered on top, plus a little bit more chilli if you fancy it and a lime wedge on the side.

quick broccoli, mushroom and sweet potato soup

feeds 2 ——— 20 minutes

1 tbsp ghee or coconut oil

100g shiitake or wild mushrooms, roughly sliced

4 spring onions, finely chopped

1 big garlic clove, finely chopped

1–2 tsp finely grated or chopped fresh ginger *(I like extra)*

1 large sweet potato or potato, scrubbed and cut into 1.5cm chunks *(about 350g)*

500ml chicken or veg stock

1 head of broccoli *(about 300g)*

2 tsp tamari or soy sauce

1 tsp fish sauce *(vegan if you prefer)* or extra tamari

A squeeze of lemon or lime juice

Sea salt and black pepper

I crave this when I'm feeling a bit run down or if I've been eating lots of rich food and when I miss my mum (and her cooking). The comforting flavours are reminiscent of a popular Filipino soup my mum used to make called *tinola*, which is packed with spring onions, garlic, ginger and soy. This quick soup is equally good with regular or sweet potatoes, and if you have any leftover cooked chicken, fish or prawns, they would be delicious warmed through at the end. I like this with chicken stock but a good-quality veg stock works well too.

———————————————————————

Melt the ghee in a medium saucepan and fry the mushrooms and most of the spring onions (save a few of the green parts for garnishing) on a medium–high heat for 4 minutes, stirring from time to time.

Add the garlic and ginger and stir-fry for about 30 seconds, swiftly followed by the sweet potato or potato chunks and the stock. Pop a lid on the pan and bring to the boil, then immediately turn down the heat to a strong simmer and cook for 10 minutes.

Use this time to chop the broccoli into small florets – bite-sized is ideal, so that you can eat this soup with a spoon. Cut off any knobbly tough bits from the stem pieces before finely slicing into rounds so that they take the same amount of time to cook as the florets.

Add the broccoli florets and stem pieces to the pan, along with the tamari/soy and fish sauce. Pop the lid on the pan and simmer strongly for 5 minutes until the sweet potato and broccoli are tender. Squeeze in a little lime or lemon juice and taste for seasoning. The tamari, stock and fish sauce will all add saltiness, so you might just want to add a little pepper rather than salt as well.

tamarind, aubergine and nut butter curry

feeds 4 ———— 40 minutes

2 tbsp coconut oil or ghee

2 medium aubergines *(500g)*, chopped into 2cm chunks

400ml tin of coconut milk

2 tsp maple syrup or coconut sugar

2 tbsp tamarind paste

700g mix of sweet potatoes and potatoes, scrubbed and chopped into 3cm chunks

300g green beans

3 tbsp smooth almond, cashew or peanut butter

Sea salt and black pepper

spice paste

1 lemongrass stalk

1 medium onion or 3 shallots, roughly chopped

1 fresh chilli, deseeded if you prefer

2 tsp ground cumin

1 tbsp garam masala

2 big garlic cloves, peeled

5cm fresh ginger *(or galangal, if you can get it)*, roughly chopped

Stalks from 1 handful of coriander

to serve

Leaves from 1 handful of coriander

4 lime wedges

Toasted cashews, roughly chopped

1 fresh chilli, chopped

I love the tanginess of the tamarind with the sweetness of coconut and the creaminess of nut butter in this hearty veg curry. Make double the spice paste and store it in the freezer so that you can use it later to make a rich noodle soup, or liven up leftover cooked rice. If pushed for time, use a Massaman or a Thai red curry paste. This is delicious served with quinoa, rice or warm flatbread or dosas.

Melt 1 tablespoon of the coconut oil in a large saucepan and fry the aubergines on a medium heat with a generous pinch of salt and pepper for 6–8 minutes, stirring from time to time.

Meanwhile, make the spice paste. Remove and discard the tough outer leaves of the lemongrass. Place in a food processor with the other paste ingredients and blitz – with a few splashes of water to get it going – until you have a chunky paste.

Once the aubergine has softened and lightly browned, transfer to a bowl. Add the remaining tablespoon of coconut oil to the pan and fry the spice paste on a low heat for 4 minutes, stirring constantly. Return the aubergine to the pan and stir to coat in the paste.

Then turn up the heat, add the coconut milk, maple syrup or coconut sugar, and tamarind paste. Fill the coconut milk tin with hot water and add that too. Add the mixed potatoes, pop a lid on the pan and cook for 15 minutes on a medium simmer.

Top the green beans (I don't bother tailing them) and slice in half at an angle, then add them to the pot with the nut butter. Give the pan a good stir and leave to simmer, uncovered, for 8 minutes until all the veg are tender when tested with a fork and the sauce has thickened and reduced a little. If the sauce is getting too thick and the veg still have a way to go, pop the lid on or add another splash of water.

Season with salt and pepper to taste, then serve in bowls with the coriander leaves, lime wedges, extra chilli and toasted cashews.

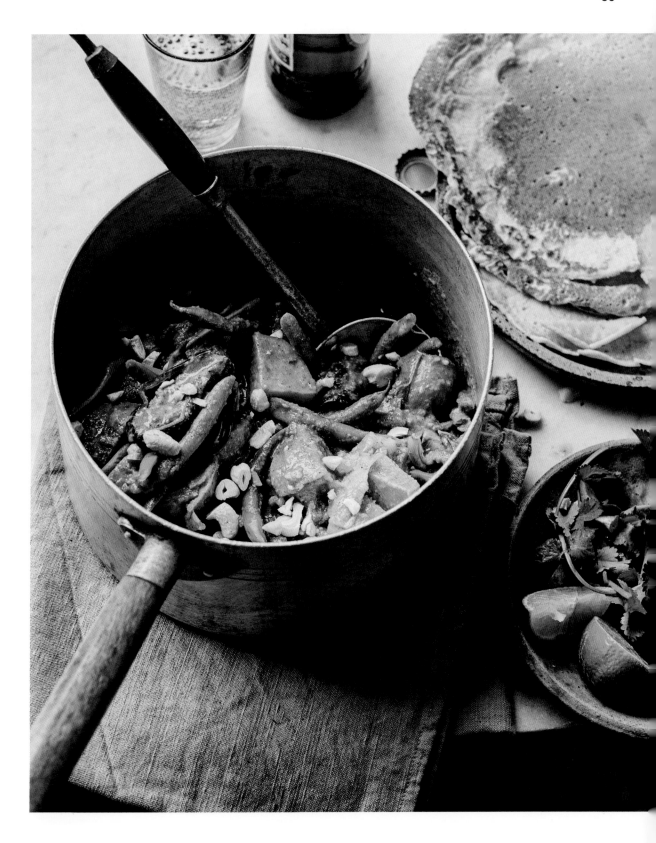

comforting bowl food

speedy chickpea and frozen kale coconut curry

feeds 2 ———— 20 minutes

1 tbsp coconut oil or ghee
½ tsp black mustard seeds
1 medium onion, diced
2 garlic cloves, finely chopped
2.5cm fresh ginger, finely grated
2 tsp ground cumin
1 tsp ground turmeric
1 tsp ground coriander
400g tin of chickpeas or other
  beans, drained and rinsed
200ml coconut milk *(½ tin –*
  see tip)
1 heaped tbsp nut butter *(such as*
  cashew or almond)
150g kale *(frozen or fresh)*
Sea salt and black pepper

optional extras
Natural yoghurt
Mango or apple chutney *(page*
  247) or tamarind chutney
Toasted nuts or seeds

I'd be very happy with a bowl of this for lunch but also with a side of quinoa or rice, with a wrap or flatbread, on toast or in a baked potato. There are lots of good shop-bought chutneys and lime pickles out there – tamarind chutney is a favourite of mine – but if your fruit bowl is groaning, why not make your own **fruit chutney** (page 247)?

Melt the coconut oil in a medium saucepan and fry the mustard seeds for 30 seconds on a medium heat, then add the onion, stirring from time to time, for 6 minutes, then add the garlic and ginger and cook for another 2 minutes.

Add the spices and a good pinch of salt and pepper and cook for a few minutes, then stir in the chickpeas. Add the coconut milk, nut butter and roughly 100ml of water, then give the pan a good stir, turn up the heat and leave to simmer on a medium heat for 5 minutes until the mixture starts to thicken and reduce.

Add the kale (roughly chopped if fresh), then cook for another 3–5 minutes (frozen greens need a bit longer) and season with salt and pepper to taste. Serve up with any of the extra toppings.

tip

Either freeze the rest of the coconut milk or include it in another dish, add it to a smoothie or use it to make a really delicious hot chocolate.

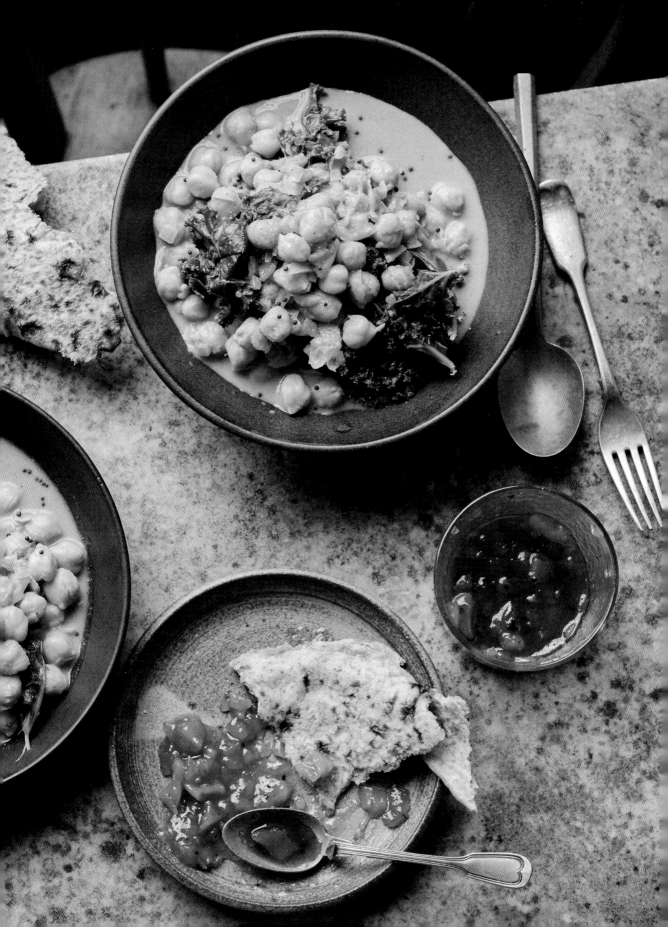

hummus bowls
with bean bites

feeds 4, makes 16 bites ———— 30 minutes

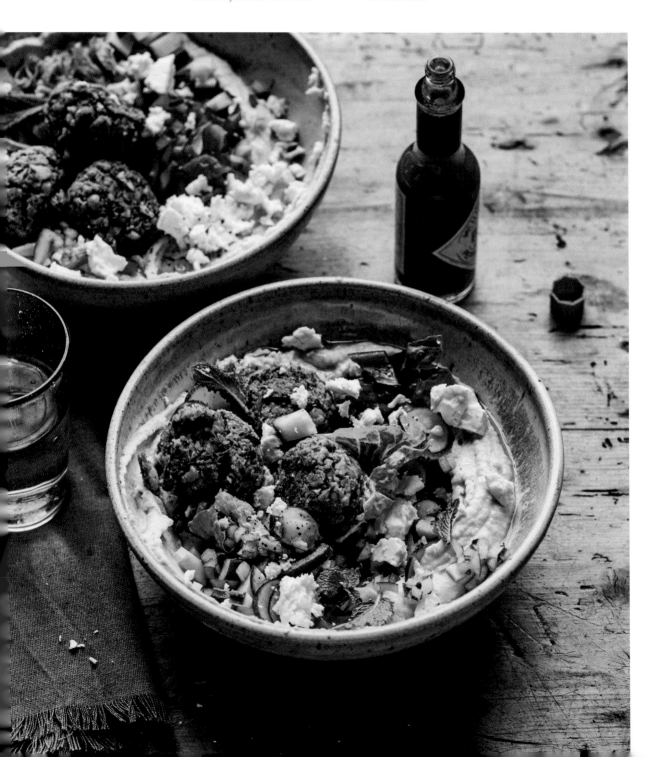

1 tbsp ghee or coconut oil

1 handful of fresh parsley or
  coriander, or a mix

400g tin of chickpeas or white
  beans, drained and rinsed

½ small onion or 4 spring onions,
  roughly chopped

2 garlic cloves, peeled

1 tsp ground cumin

Grated zest of 1 lemon

1 tsp baking powder

2 tbsp flour *(plain, buckwheat
  or chickpea/gram)*, plus extra
  if needed

Sea salt and black pepper

hummus

400g tin of white beans
  (I like butter beans) or chickpeas,
  drained and rinsed

3½ tbsp tahini *(stirred well in the
  jar first)*

1 large garlic clove, peeled

Juice of 1 lemon

A drizzle of extra-virgin olive
  or chilli oil

A pinch of ground cumin
  (optional)

optional extras

Lettuce or other salad leaves

4 lemon wedges

Sliced cucumber, red pepper,
  tomatoes or radishes

Crumbled feta or fried halloumi
  or 2 hard-boiled eggs, quartered

Spicy sauce

Pickled onion *(page 246)* or
  chopped spring onions

When you can't get fresh falafel from a falafel master, this is the next best thing. I love them made with chickpeas but, for variety, here's a delicious version where you can switch chickpeas for beans, if you like. Delicious hot or cold, and lovely pan-fried or baked, for ease. Keep any leftover mix in the fridge for up to a week to make and fry them from scratch, or just reheat any leftovers by dry frying them in a pan on a medium heat.

Preheat the oven to fan 220°C/gas mark 7, place the ghee on a large baking tray and pop it in the oven to heat up.

Meanwhile, blitz the herbs briefly in a food processor for 30 seconds, then add all the other bean-bite ingredients to the food processor – except for the baking powder and flour – and blitz until still chunky. Season with salt and pepper.

Take the food processor bowl off the stand and remove the blade, then sprinkle in the baking powder with ½ teaspoon of salt and lots of black pepper. Add the flour a tablespoon at a time; if the mixture is sticky, it may need a touch more flour. Try a little of the mix and add more salt and pepper if needed, as the extra flour may need more seasoning.

Form the mixture into 16 balls (each roughly the size of a golf ball), then place on the prepared baking tray and bake for 16 minutes, carefully turning them after about 9 minutes to get a lightly golden colour on each side. After 16 minutes they'll still feel soft – leave to cool for 10 minutes before serving and they'll firm up.

While they're cooking, add all the hummus ingredients to the food processor – except the oil and cumin – no need to clean it out first. Blitz until smooth, adding a tablespoon of water as you go. Season with salt and pepper to taste, then transfer to four bowls and add a drizzle of olive or chilli oil and a tiny sprinkling of cumin, if you like.

Add your choice of optional extras to each bowl and tuck in when the bean bites are ready.

cosy coconut lentils with kachumber

feeds 6 ——— 30 minutes

2 tsp cumin seeds or 1 tbsp
  ground cumin
1 tsp black mustard seeds
1 tsp fennel seeds
1 tsp ground turmeric
2 tbsp coconut oil or ghee
1 large onion, finely chopped
3 garlic cloves, finely chopped
4cm fresh ginger, finely chopped
  or grated
A pinch of chilli flakes or a little
  chopped fresh chilli
500g red lentils, rinsed
400ml tin of coconut milk
2 handfuls of fresh coriander,
  stalks finely chopped
1 litre veg or chicken stock
Sea salt and black pepper

kachumber

2 handfuls of deseeded cucumber
  chunks
2 handfuls of ripe tomato chunks
¼ small red onion, chopped into
  chunks, or 3 spring onions
¼ tsp ground cumin
1 tbsp lemon or lime juice
2 tbsp extra-virgin olive oil
1 fresh green chilli, deseeded and
  chopped, or a pinch of chilli flakes
1 small handful of mint leaves

to serve

Natural or coconut yoghurt
Pickled onion *(page 246)*
Leaves from 2 handfuls of
  fresh coriander

Enjoy this dish just as it is, or nice and thick with quinoa, rice, a wrap or a baked potato, or go soupier, with more stock. I purposefully make extra so I have leftovers. Once the lentils have cooled, they will thicken, so when you reheat, add half a mug of water per portion and stir it in as the lentils warm through. Kachumber is a refreshing salad in its own right, delicious with soups and curries, or chopped finely, used as a salsa. Use ripe tomatoes – it will make all the difference.

In a large saucepan, toast the cumin, mustard and fennel seeds on a medium heat for a minute until they start to pop. (If using ground cumin, include it later with the turmeric.)

Add the coconut oil, onion and a little salt, then turn up the heat and fry for 8 minutes, stirring every now and then. Add the garlic, ginger, chilli, turmeric and ground cumin, if using, and fry for another few minutes.

Next, add the lentils, coconut milk, chopped coriander stalks and stock. Stir everything together, then turn up the heat to high, pop a lid on the pan and simmer on a medium heat for 12 minutes. Give it a good stir every now and then, stirring right to the bottom of the pan to make sure the lentils don't catch on the base.

Meanwhile, make the kachumber. Simply toss together all of the ingredients in a bowl with a pinch of sea salt, taste, and leave to one side until ready to serve.

Once the lentils are tender, season with salt and pepper to taste, then serve topped with some yoghurt, pickled onion and the coriander leaves, with the kachumber on the side.

feel good

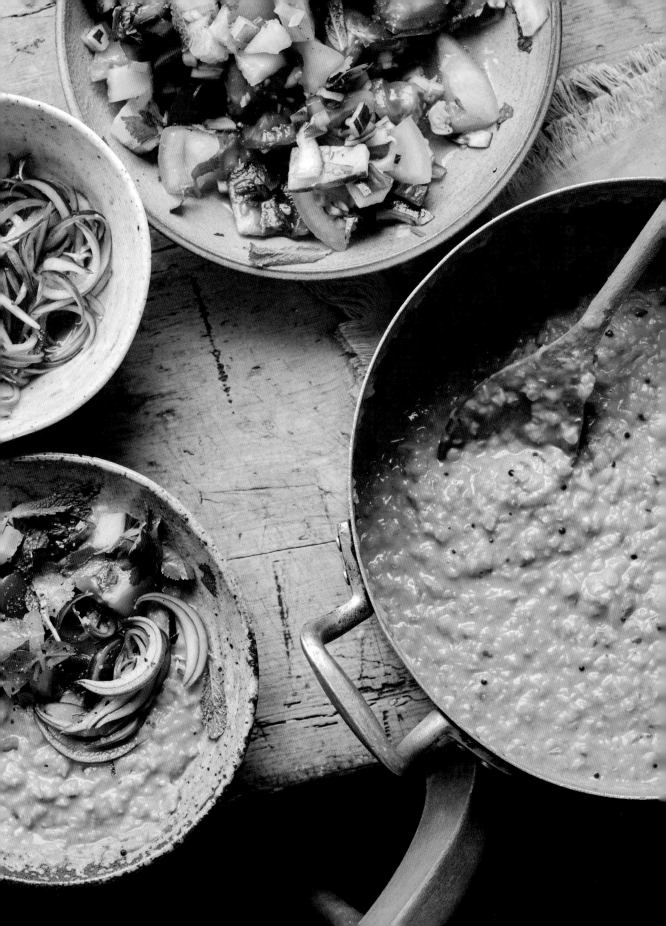

any bean, any lentil chilli

feeds 5 ——— 45 minutes

1 ½ tbsp ghee or olive oil
2 onions, finely chopped
2 large handfuls of diced veg
(such as carrots, peppers, celery
or courgettes)
3 garlic cloves, finely chopped
2 tbsp tomato purée
400g tin of chopped tomatoes
180g uncooked green or brown
lentils, rinsed
600ml veg stock
2 × 400g tins of mixed beans,
drained and rinsed
1 tsp maple syrup (optional)
Sea salt and black pepper

spices and herbs

1 tbsp ground cumin or 1 ½ tsp
cumin seeds
A pinch of chilli flakes/powder
or cayenne pepper
1 ½ tsp smoked paprika
½ tsp ground cinnamon
1 heaped tsp dried oregano

limey cabbage and onions

4 handfuls of finely shredded
red cabbage
1 small red onion, finely sliced
Juice of 1 lime

optional extras

Natural yoghurt or soured cream
Grated Cheddar
Fresh coriander
Pickled sliced jalapeños, deseeded
if you prefer

A chilli to feed your street! This is so easy and makes five portions, so you can happily cook a big batch and freeze any extra for another day. I prefer green lentils for this dish, but brown lentils are good too. Work with whatever spices you've got and amp up the spice levels as much as you like – I've gone for a gentler mix, so that you can use it for the whole family. This is a real favourite of mine.

Melt the ghee in a big saucepan, add the onions and a pinch of salt and fry on a medium heat for 5 minutes.

Add the diced veg and fry for 2 minutes, then add the garlic, spices and herbs, and stir-fry for another 2–3 minutes, stirring occasionally and adding a splash of water if any of the ingredients start to stick.

Add the tomato purée and let it cook for a minute or so, stirring it regularly so that it darkens in colour. Add the tinned tomatoes, lentils and stock. Bring to the boil, then reduce the heat to medium, pop a lid on the pan and simmer for 15 minutes. Stir every 5 minutes or so, making sure you get to the bottom of the pan so the lentils don't stick. Add more hot water if needed.

Meanwhile, make the limey cabbage and onions by mixing all the ingredients together. Add a good pinch of salt, toss everything together well and leave to quickly 'pickle'.

Add the tinned beans to the chilli, turn up the heat and simmer strongly for another 10 minutes with the lid off, so the sauce can thicken and reduce.

Once the veg and lentils are nicely tender, season the chilli with salt and pepper to taste, adding the maple syrup if you like. Remove from the heat and divide between bowls, top with a generous spoonful of the limey cabbage and onions and serve with the optional extras.

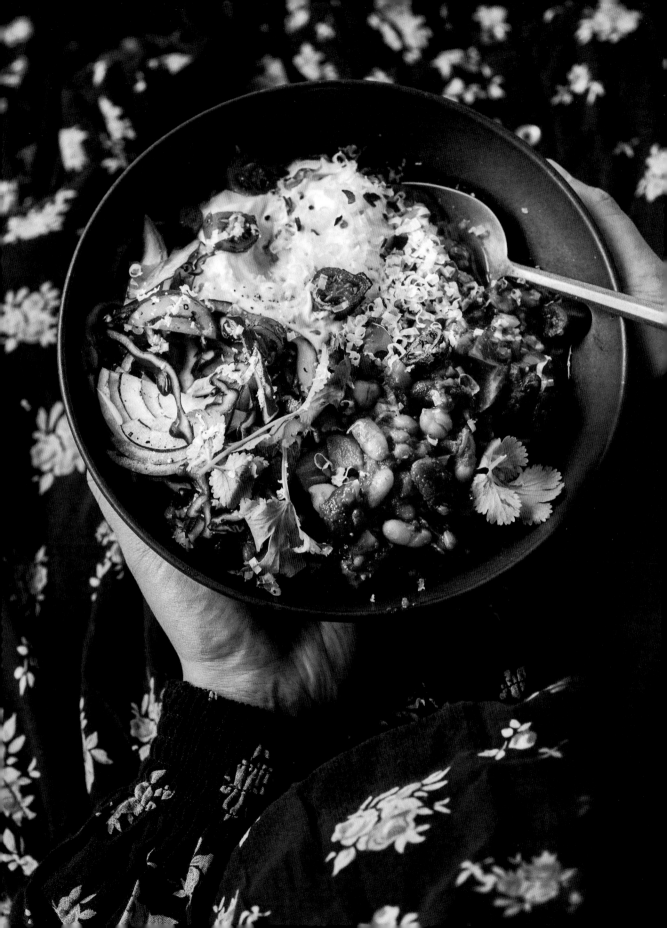

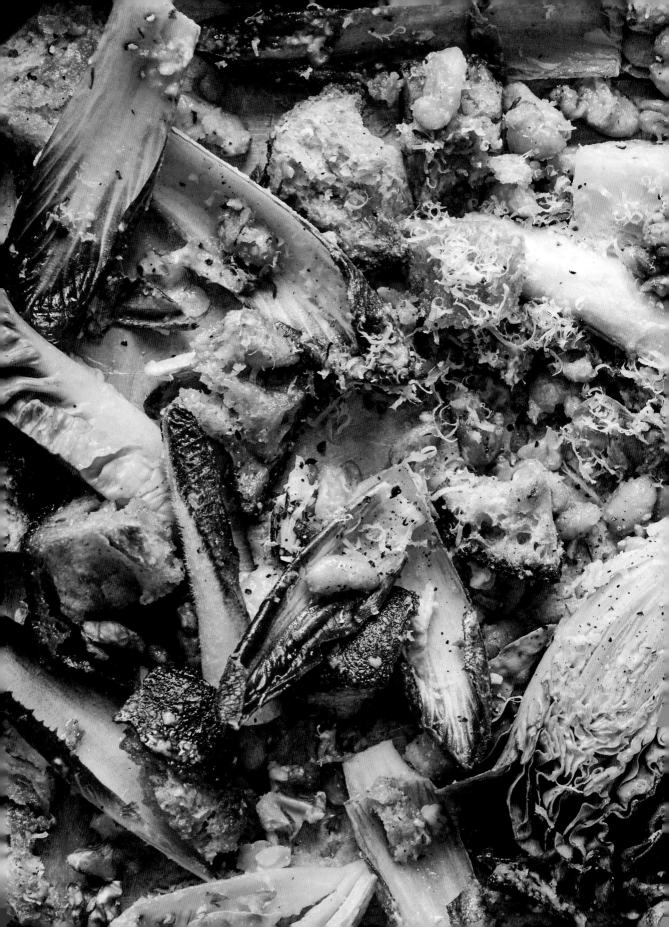

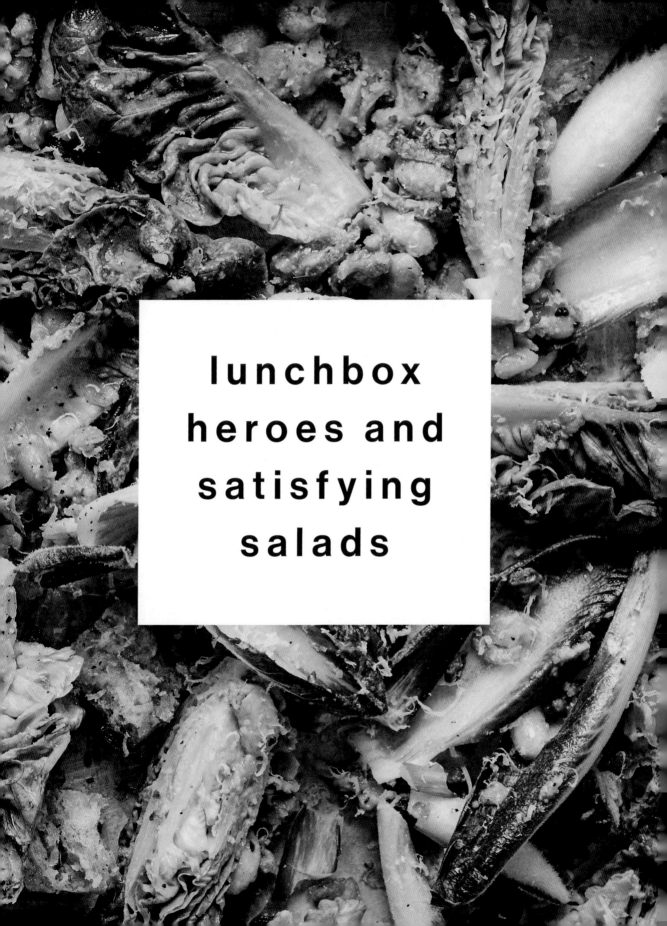

lunchbox
heroes and
satisfying
salads

/ what makes a salad satisfying? /

What makes a salad satisfying? For me, it's a balance of hot and cold, some heartiness and some lighter, fresher elements, with a combination of fantastic flavours and contrasting textures from nuts, seeds, grains, beans, herbs and lots of veg, both raw and roasted. Delicious dressings, drizzles, sauces and bright pickles are also key to bringing salads to life and taking them to the next level, flavour-wise. You'll find them scattered throughout the chapter – including a **carrot-ginger dressing** (page 85), a **garlicky, herbacous chimichurri drizzle** (page 90) and a **spicy, miso-based Korean-inspired sauce** (page 72) – and turn to pages 246–7 for a few of my favourite pickles and the **Freestyle Fruit-Bowl Chutney**.

Among my lunchbox heroes are recipes that travel well, hence they are perfect for packing up for work lunches – hopefully a 'laptop-free lunch' allowing you to take a break from your desk to enjoy a few moments of peace on a busy day. If you haven't done so already, get yourself some good-quality lidded containers and maybe a flask for soups and stews. That way you'll always have a delicious portable lunch to look forward to – something to help spur you on through the morning and then power you through the afternoon.

I especially love the **Roasted White Beans with Caesar-style Tahini Dressing** (page 76), while the **Sweet Potato Salad with Spicy Peanut-Lime Sauce** (page 102) makes a great lunchbox option. A special shout-out for the **Quick Leeky Beans** (page 94), a different way to do beans on toast, and don't miss the plant-based **'chuna'** (smashed chickpeas to replace tinned tuna) salad on page 86 – delicious in a wrap for lunch when you're out and about or in a baked potato to enjoy at home. It really hits the spot as a veggie alternative to a childhood classic.

For other lunchbox ideas, see the **Comforting Bowl Food** chapter on pages 36–87.

mixed quinoa bowl
with red miso sauce

feeds 2 ———— 20 minutes

1 tbsp ghee or coconut oil
250g mushrooms, roughly sliced
2 tsp toasted sesame oil
250g cooked quinoa *(about 100g uncooked)*
2+ eggs
1 head of broccoli or 1 large handful of green beans
Sea salt and black pepper

red miso sauce *makes double*
2 tbsp red miso paste
1 tbsp mirin
1½ tbsp tamari or soy sauce
2 garlic cloves, peeled
2 tbsp maple syrup *(or to taste)*
1 fresh red chilli or pinch of chilli flakes *(to taste)*

to serve
2 tbsp sesame seeds
2 tbsp kimchi

optional extras
1 large carrot or ⅓ cucumber, peeled into ribbons with a vegetable peeler
A few sliced radishes or pickled radishes *(page 246)*
Sliced spring onions
Crumbled dried seaweed

Inspired by the Korean dish *bibimbap*, this is a delicious way to DIY things at home with mixed veg and eggs on top. The cooked quinoa is fried in a little toasted sesame oil so you get crispy golden bits, but you could also use leftover rice. These bowls are fast to make – a great option to serve a crowd – with lots of satisfying contrast from the hot and cold ingredients, the golden-edged mushrooms and tangy and refreshing toppings like kimchi. Serve with raw crunchy fresh veg or **Quick-pickled Veg** (page 246) or a bit of both.

Place the ingredients for the sauce in the small bowl of a food processor, then blitz to a paste and taste for seasoning.

Melt the ghee in a large frying pan, add the mushrooms and fry in a single layer on a medium heat for about 4 minutes until golden, then turn over and fry on the other side until golden all over. Push the mushrooms right over to one side of the frying pan, add the toasted sesame oil and fry the cooked quinoa in a single layer, undisturbed, for about 5 minutes, then turn and repeat. Season the quinoa and mushrooms with salt and pepper.

Meanwhile, cook the eggs in a pan of boiling salted water on a medium simmer for 7 minutes, then remove and peel once cool enough to handle. Chop the broccoli into bite-sized florets and finely slice the stem, or if you're using green beans, top (but don't tail) them and cut into thirds. Add the broccoli or beans to the same pan of water and cook on a medium simmer for 5 minutes until tender.

Serve up the quinoa and mushrooms with the veg, add a boiled egg and drizzle a few tablespoons of the sauce over each bowl. Scatter over the sesame seeds, kimchi and any of the optional extras you like.

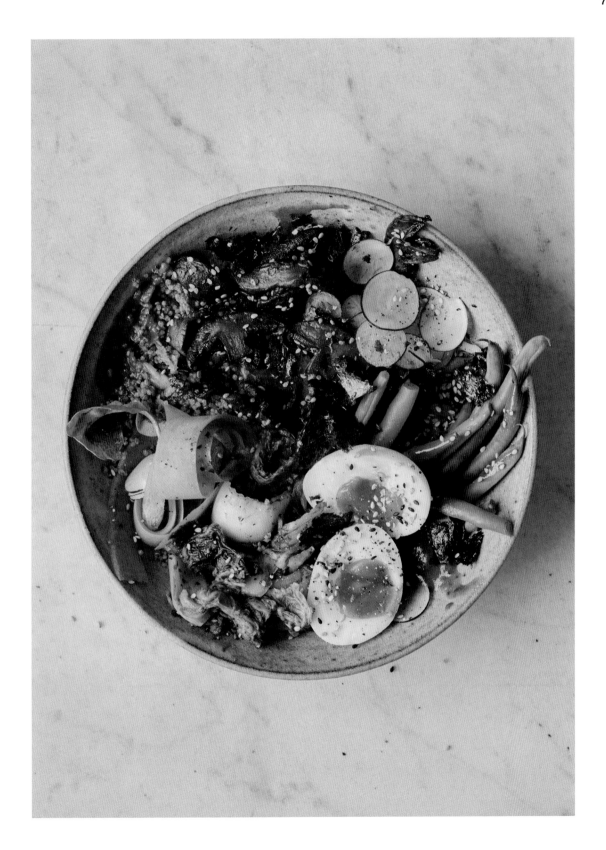

lunchbox heroes and satisfying salads

winter salad with citrus-maple-ginger dressing

Feeds 4, or 8 as part of a spread ——— 30 minutes

80g whole almonds
250g tricolour quinoa, rinsed
500ml veg stock
40g dried fruit *(such as sour berries, cranberries or raisins)*
2 handfuls of fresh parsley, roughly chopped
2 handfuls of rocket or baby spinach, roughly chopped
100g goat's cheese or feta, crumbled at the end *(optional)*

roast veg

2 tbsp ghee or olive oil
800g squash *(unpeeled)*, deseeded and chopped into wedges
1 large red onion, cut into wedges
1 tbsp balsamic vinegar
Sea salt and black pepper

citrus-maple-ginger dressing

4 tbsp extra-virgin olive oil
1 tbsp balsamic vinegar
3 tbsp fresh lemon or orange juice and 1 tsp grated zest
1 garlic clove, finely chopped
15g ginger, grated to give 1½ tsp juice *(see tip)*

tip

Use the leftover grated ginger pulp in a stir-fry or make ginger tea.

This is a super-adaptable seasonal salad, made here with tricolour quinoa, though it would be equally good with buckwheat, plain quinoa, brown or wild rice, Puy lentils or a mixture, bearing in mind that cooking times will vary. When I'm making this for friends, I use a combination of beautiful delicata squash and trusty butternut squash, though you could use any type. I don't peel the squash unless it has a very thick skin.

Preheat the oven to fan 220°C/gas mark 9, then place the ghee in a large roasting tray and pop in the oven to heat up.

Carefully toss the squash and onion in the hot ghee with the balsamic vinegar. Season with salt and pepper, spread out in a single layer and roast for 15 minutes, then gently toss in the tray and roast for another 10 minutes until tender and golden around the edges.

Meanwhile, pop the almonds in a second roasting tray and toast for 5–10 minutes until golden, keeping an eye on them so they don't burn. Tip out onto a chopping board, then roughly chop and set aside.

Cook the quinoa in the stock for 18–20 minutes (or according to the packet instructions) until tender, then leave to stand for 5 minutes off the heat, with a lid on the pan. Fluff with a fork, making sure all the liquid has evaporated (drain any excess), and set aside to cool.

Mix the dressing ingredients together in a big serving bowl and season to taste with salt and pepper.

Add all the other salad ingredients to the bowl (keeping back some almonds and herbs for garnishing), then tip in the quinoa and toss together. Add the squash and onions, gently toss everything together and serve topped with a final flourish of almonds and herbs.

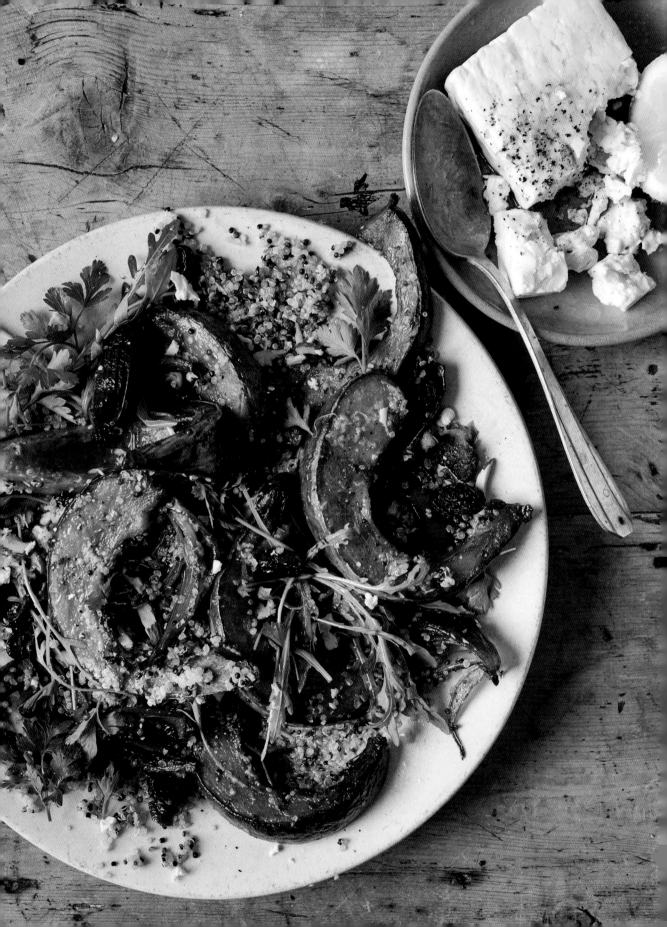

roasted white beans with Caesar-style tahini dressing

feeds 2–3 as a main or 4 as a side ——— 40 minutes

3 tbsp ghee or olive oil

400g tin of white beans or chickpeas, drained and rinsed

1 tsp dried thyme or rosemary

1 handful of walnuts or pecans

1 handful of bread, cut into 1cm chunks

1 Little Gem lettuce

1 head of red chicory or another Little Gem lettuce

Sea salt and black pepper

tahini dressing *makes extra*

2 anchovy fillets *(from a jar or tin)*

2½ tbsp tahini *(stirred well in the the jar first)*

1 garlic clove

¾ tsp Dijon mustard

2 tbsp extra-virgin olive oil

3 tbsp lemon juice

1 handful of grated Parmesan or other hard cheese, plus extra to serve

variation

To make this plant-based, swap the anchovies for 1 teaspoon of vegan Worcestershire sauce or 1 teaspoon of miso paste plus 2 teaspoons of pickling liquid from a jar of capers. Instead of cheese, use 1 teaspoon of nutritional yeast. Use olive oil rather than ghee.

Use any crunchy salad leaves you like here, but I particularly love the combination of Gem lettuce and red chicory for the contrast in colour and between the sweeter and more bitter leaves. I love this dressing, so this recipe makes lots – you'll have extra. Use it as a dip, in a lunch wrap the next day, on roasted cauliflower and broccoli, drizzled over grilled sweet potatoes or tossed through a pasta salad. The croutons are a great way to use up bread that is going stale.

Preheat the oven to fan 220°C/gas mark 9, then place 1½ tablespoons of the ghee in a large roasting tray and pop in the oven to heat up.

Meanwhile, dry the beans well in a tea towel to ensure they don't spit in the hot ghee.

Once the tray is hot, remove from the oven and toss the beans in the melted ghee, along with a good pinch of salt and pepper and the dried herbs, then spread out in a single layer and roast for 15 minutes. Add the rest of ghee and the nuts and bread chunks, toss everything together well and spread out again into a single layer, then pop back in the oven to cook for another 10 minutes. Remove the tray from the oven and let the roasted bean mixture cool for 10 minutes, if you've got time, as it will crisp up more as it cools.

Meanwhile, add the dressing ingredients to the small bowl of a food processor, along with about 4 tablespoons of water, then blitz to combine. Season with salt and pepper and add 1–2 tablespoons of water if the dressing needs thinning down.

Slice off the ends of the lettuces and separate the leaves, then wash and dry really well so that the dressing doesn't slide off the leaves. Arrange haphazardly on a big serving platter.

Scatter the roasted bean mixture over the leaves, drizzle over half of the dressing and sprinkle with extra grated cheese.

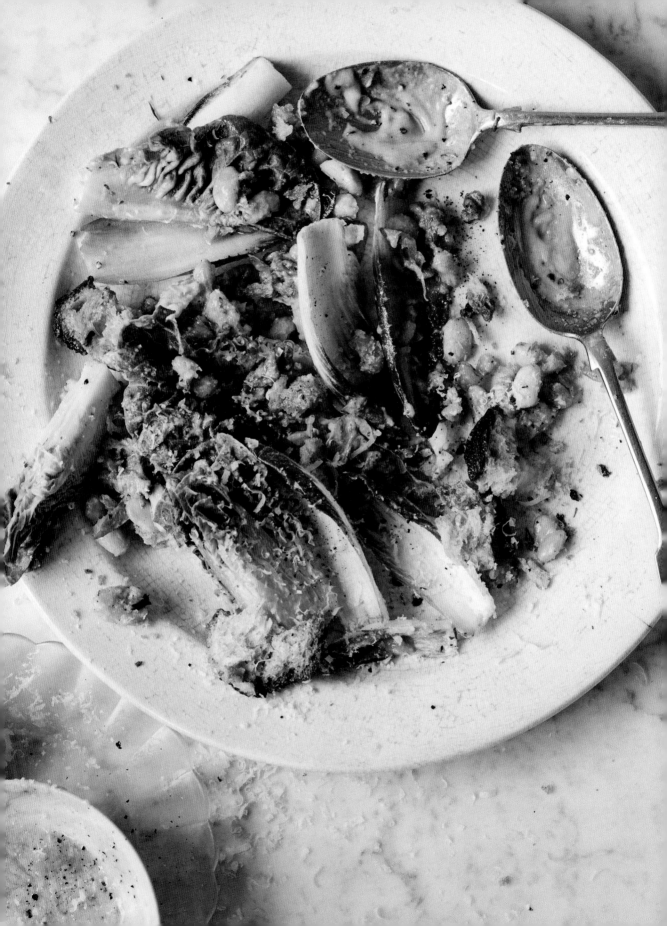

baked feta and ras el hanout broccoli salad

feeds 2 as a main ——— 30 minutes

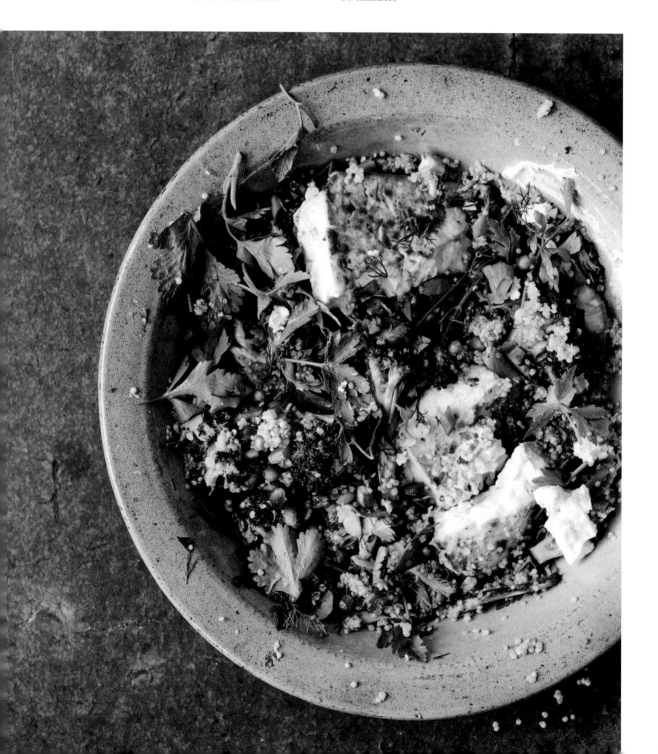

1 tbsp ghee or coconut oil

1 large head of broccoli

2 tsp ras el hanout spice *(see introduction)*, plus extra to serve

200g block of feta, drained and sliced in half

150g quinoa, rinsed

300ml veg stock

3 tbsp extra-virgin olive oil

Juice of 1 lemon and 1 tsp zest

2 spring onions, chopped

1 big handful of pomegranate seeds or chopped tomatoes

2 handfuls of fresh coriander or parsley, finely chopped

1 small handful of fresh mint or dill, finely chopped

Sea salt and black pepper

Here's a beautiful roasted broccoli and feta salad that would also be wonderful with cauliflower. The Moroccan spice mix ras el hanout can also be swapped for baharat spice mix or harissa. Alternatively, make your own from ½ teaspoon each of ground cumin and coriander and ¼ teaspoon each of smoked paprika, cinnamon, turmeric and cardamom or ginger. Don't worry if you haven't got them all – use what you have to hand to make your own unique mix.

Preheat the oven to fan 220°C/gas mark 9, then place the ghee on a large baking tray and pop in the oven to heat up.

Chop the broccoli into small florets and slice up the stem. Once the tray is hot, remove from the oven and toss the broccoli in the melted ghee with 1½ teaspoons of ras el hanout and a good pinch of salt and pepper, then spread out in an even layer – using tongs to help, if you have them – leaving two gaps for each half of the feta. Add the feta, sprinkle the remaining ras el hanout on top and roast for 12 minutes. Remove from the oven, toss the broccoli in the tray, being careful not to disturb the feta, and roast for another 8–10 minutes until the broccoli is tender and going golden at the edges.

Meanwhile, cook the quinoa in the stock in a medium saucepan, with a lid on (according to the packet instructions) or until all the liquid has been absorbed. Remove from the hob and leave to sit for 4 minutes off the heat, then take off the lid and fluff the quinoa with a fork.

Make the dressing by whisking the olive oil and lemon juice and zest with a fork in a large wide bowl or platter, then add the cooked quinoa and toss in the dressing, which it will absorb as it cools. Toss through all the remaining fresh ingredients and season with salt and pepper to taste.

Chop the cooked broccoli so that it is bite-sized, then toss with the rest of the salad. Top with the baked feta and enjoy straight away while the cheese is hot. Sprinkle a little extra spice on top of the baked feta to finish, if you like.

variation

Swap the feta for roasted butter beans for a plant-based version – you will still get golden edges and a creamy buttery centre. Use coconut oil rather than ghee.

fennel and orange harissa-chickpea salad

feeds 4 as a side ——— 15 minutes

400g tin of chickpeas, drained,
   rinsed and dried well
3 tsp *(rose)* harissa paste
4 tbsp extra-virgin olive oil
Juice of 1 small lemon
1 handful of walnuts or almonds
   (about 30g)
1 ripe orange or blood orange
1 large fennel bulb
2 handfuls of olives *(120g pitted
   and ideally the black wrinkly kind)*
2 big handfuls of fresh parsley
   leaves or mixed mint and parsley
200g feta, roughly crumbled
Sea salt and black pepper
2 tsp sumac or grated lemon zest,
   to serve *(optional)*

This gorgeous salad brings back incredible memories of a spring week in New York. One of my favourite food magazines, **Cherry Bombe**, was holding its annual festival and, together with fellow chefs Hetty McKinnon, Anna Jones and Maxine Thompson, we made hundreds of portions of this salad. It takes minutes and is packed with flavour – heaven on a plate! Orange and fennel is a classic combination; even if you're wary of fruit in salads, do give it a go. If you want to turn this into a main, it would be delicious with roasted sweet potatoes or a grilled oily fish like mackerel.

Place the chickpeas in a bowl with the harissa, olive oil, lemon juice and some salt and pepper, then mix together well and set aside.

Toast the walnuts or almonds in a frying pan on a medium heat for 3 minutes, tossing halfway through, then very roughly chop them.

Prepare the orange by peeling and removing the pith and any pips before slicing into segments – don't worry if the segments aren't perfect. For the fennel, slice in half lengthways, then finely slice and save the delicate fennel fronds for garnishing.

Place the orange segments and fennel on a serving platter, add the chickpeas and all the remaining ingredients, reserving some of the feta, and toss everything together. Finish by garnishing with the reserved feta and fennel fronds, sprinkling with the sumac or lemon zest, if using, and scattering over the nuts.

Spanish-style salad

feeds 2–3 as a main or 6 as a side ———— 15 minutes

8 asparagus spears, ends
  snapped off
3 eggs
1 handful of olives *(ideally the
  green Spanish ones)*
2 smoked mackerel or smoked
  trout fillets
2 handfuls of tinned sweetcorn
1 small onion, finely sliced into rings
3 ripe tomatoes, sliced into wedges
2 large carrots, scrubbed and
  roughly grated
4 handfuls of torn lettuce
Sea salt and black pepper

dressing

5 tbsp extra-virgin olive oil
2 tbsp red wine vinegar

Fresh, crunchy and full of colour, *ensalada mixta* is traditionally made with tuna. I've gone for smoked mackerel here, but tinned sardines or anchovies would work or swap the fish for artichoke hearts. In Spain, I've had this with white asparagus, but as a nod to the delicious British variety, I've used green. To make this even heartier, toss it with a few handfuls of cooked potatoes or lentils. And as my friend Kitty – who styled this book and whose heart is in Mallorca – says, it's the red wine vinegar that makes this!

Bring a medium pan of salted water to the boil and cook the asparagus for 3–4 minutes, depending on thickness, then scoop out with tongs or a slotted spoon and place on a serving platter.

Carefully drop the eggs into the boiling water in the pan and cook for 8 minutes until hard-boiled. Cool under cold running water and then peel and slice into quarters.

Meanwhile, make the dressing by whisking together the oil and vinegar and seasoning with salt and pepper to taste.

Add all the other ingredients to the serving platter, along with the boiled eggs, then gently toss in the dressing and serve straight away.

smoked mackerel pâté

feeds 2 ——— 10 minutes

3 smoked mackerel fillets *(190g)*
2 tbsp lemon juice and a little
    grated zest
6 tbsp Greek-style yoghurt
2 spring onions
1 handful of fresh parsley
Sea salt and black pepper

to serve
Toast
A big pile of watercress
½ cucumber, sliced into rounds
A few radishes, thinly sliced

optional extras
1 ripe tomato, sliced
Pickled onion *(page 246)* or
    Quick-pickled Veg *(page 246)*
Gherkins or capers
1 tsp creamed horseradish
Celery leaves

A speedy lunch or a crowd-pleasing party bite. Serve with toast or crackers, a big platter of crudités like fennel or carrots, or simply spread on rounds of cucumber. Check out my other favourite spread, **Sun-dried Tomato Tapenade**, on page 215. This pâté is also delicious made with smoked trout.

Roughly chop all the ingredients for the pâté, and mix together with a generous pinch of salt and pepper. (I like to include the skin of the smoked mackerel, but leave out if you prefer.) Keep back a few herbs for garnishing later. Taste for seasoning and adjust if needed.

Enjoy straight away or place in a covered bowl and pop in the fridge for a few hours.

Serve on toast (I like rye toast) with the watercress, cucumber and radishes, plus any of the optional extras. Garnish with the reserved herbs.

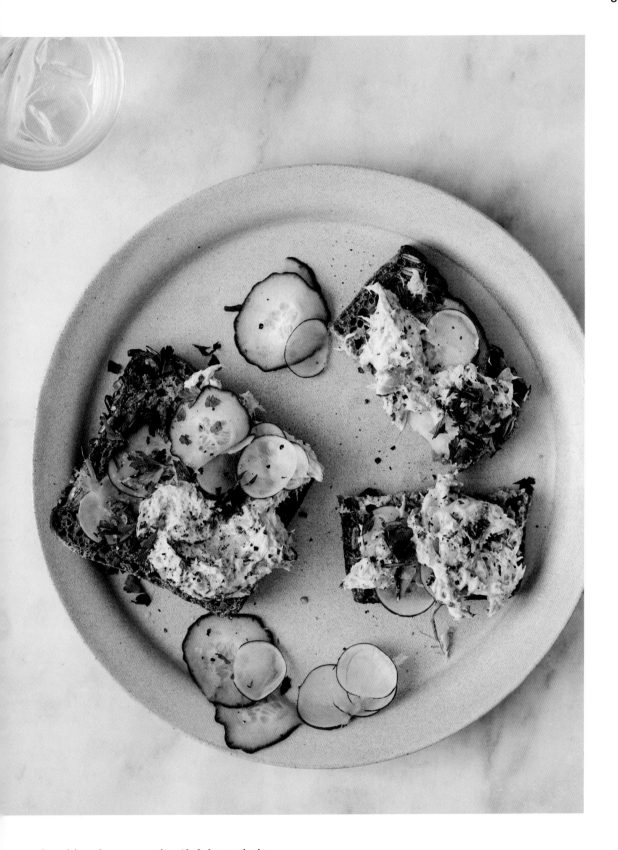

lunchbox heroes and satisfying salads

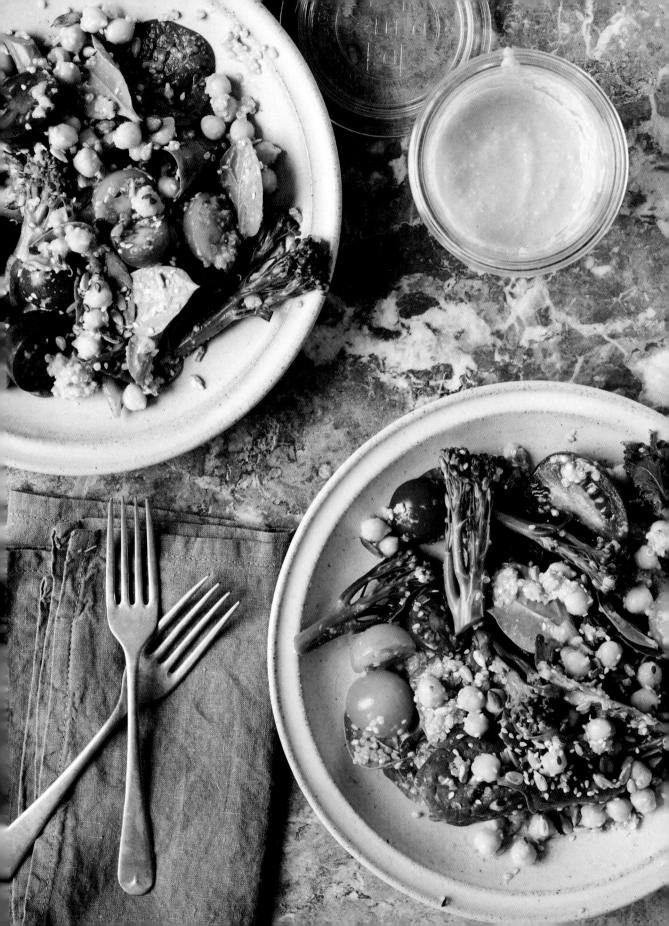

big broccoli and spinach salad with carrot-ginger dressing

feeds 2 ———— 15 minutes *(25 minutes if cooking the quinoa)*

1 large handful of bite-sized
  broccoli florets, stems sliced thinly
100g baby spinach
400g tin of chickpeas, drained,
  rinsed and dried
1 handful of cherry tomatoes
  (I like a mix of colours), halved
About 150g cooked quinoa or
  brown rice *(about 80g uncooked
  – see tip)*
1 handful of seeds *(such as
  pumpkin or sunflower)*, toasted,
  to serve

dressing *makes extra*
2 medium carrots, scrubbed
  (about 200g)
2 tbsp chopped fresh ginger
3½ tbsp extra-virgin olive oil
1 tbsp toasted sesame oil
½ small white onion or
  3 spring onions
3 tbsp rice vinegar or apple
  cider vinegar
2½ tbsp white miso paste
Sea salt

A favourite lunchbox salad of mine, and happily this makes extra dressing, so drizzle over roast veg and noodles. I love carrot-ginger soup in the winter, and carrot-ginger dressing is one of my go-tos in the warmer months. It's inspired by a Japanese dressing, the white miso paste giving it a beautifully salty-sweet umami flavour. Swap the cooked chickpeas for lentils or other beans, if you like.

———————————————————————————

Steam the broccoli for 4–5 minutes in a small pan until just tender. You can do this by putting a small amount of water with a little pinch of salt in a pan so that it covers the bottom by about half an inch, and cooking the broccoli in it with a lid on the pan.

Place all the ingredients for the dressing – except the salt – in a high-powdered blender or a food processor and blend until smooth, then season with salt to taste. If your blender isn't high-powered, roughly grate the carrots and ginger first before adding them to the blender with the rest of the ingredients. Add about 4 tablespoons of water to the dressing to make it drizzly; it is a thick dressing, but add more water to thin it out further if you fancy.

Toss all the salad ingredients together, drizzle over about half of the dressing and scatter over the seeds. Serve any extra dressing on the side and keep the rest in a clean screw-top jar in the fridge.

tip

To prepare the quinoa from scratch, cook it following the packet instructions and, in the last 4 minutes, add the broccoli florets to sit on top. Remove from the heat and leave the lid on for 3 minutes.

lunchbox 'chuna' ~ two ways

feeds 2 ———— 10 minutes

400g tin of chickpeas, drained
  and rinsed
2 spring onions or ¼ red onion,
  finely chopped
3 mixed handfuls of finely diced
  celery, red pepper and carrot
2 tbsp capers, chopped gherkins,
  pickles or olives, plus 1 tbsp
  brine from the jar
1 ½ tbsp mayonnaise *(vegan if you
  prefer)* or thick natural yoghurt
Juice of ½ lemon or 1 ½ tbsp
  apple cider vinegar
½ tsp dried dill or a sprinkling of
  chopped fresh dill or parsley
1 tsp mustard *(any kind)*
2 tsp curry powder *(optional)*
Sea salt and black pepper
2 big handfuls of lettuce leaves,
  to serve

optional extras

2 tbsp tinned or smoked fish or
  a chopped hard-boiled egg
A little chopped fresh chilli *(such
  as jalapeño)* or spicy sauce

A favourite fast packed lunch. Inspired by tuna sandwiches from my childhood, this chickpea version, nicknamed 'chuna' by the plant-based community, is really tasty and quick. Enjoy it 'two ways' by trying the curried chickpea version. It's a great way to pack lots of crunchy fresh veg in at lunchtime. On colder days, I like it 'tuna melt' style in a toasted sandwich or stuffed into a jacket or roasted sweet potato. Also delicious in a wrap or with more greens as a salad. Most of the time, I just eat it straight out the bowl.

In a medium bowl, roughly mash half of the chickpeas with a fork or with a potato masher if you have one.

Add all the other ingredients to the bowl, apart from the lettuce, including the curry powder if making curried chuna. Toss to combine and taste for seasoning.

Pack in a lunchbox or divide between plates or bowls and serve with the lettuce and any of the optional extras.

tip

Try making this in advance or make extra, as it gets even tastier the next day.

feel good

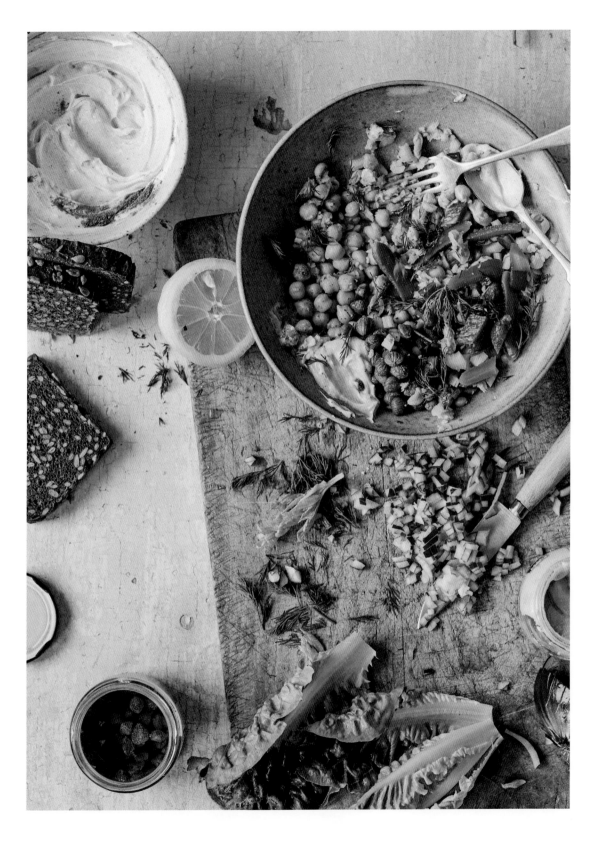

lunchbox heroes and satisfying salads

lunchbox orzo pasta salad

feeds 4 ——— 45 minutes

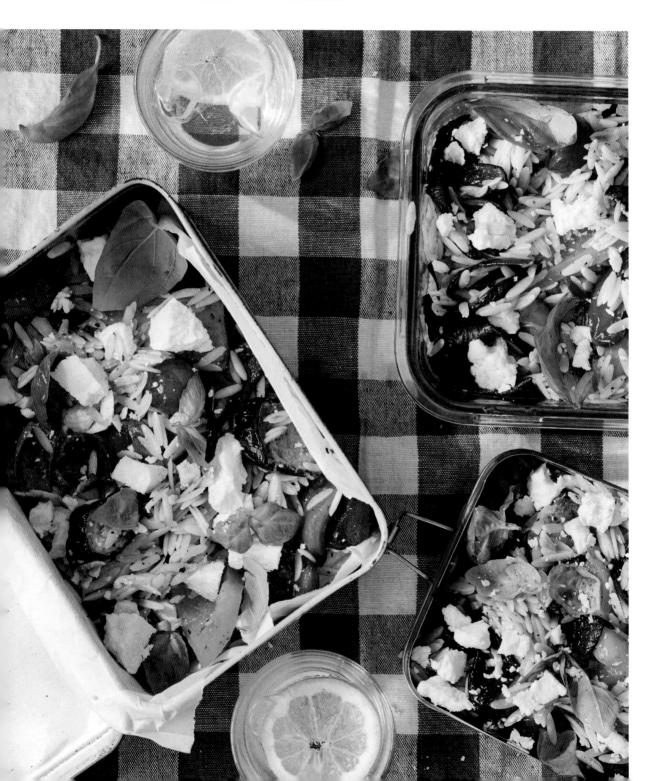

2 tbsp olive oil or ghee

2 peppers *(red, orange or yellow)*, deseeded and cut into 1.5cm chunks

2 courgettes, cut into 1.5cm chunks

1 red onion, roughly chopped

1 tsp dried oregano

2 garlic cloves, roughly chopped

200g dried orzo pasta

Sea salt and black pepper

dressing

Juice of 1 small lemon and a little grated zest

4 tbsp extra-virgin olive oil

1 tsp dried oregano

1 garlic clove, finely chopped

A little pinch of chilli flakes

to serve

2 handfuls of basil, leaves torn and stems finely chopped

1 handful of cherry tomatoes, halved, or 1 handful of sun-dried tomatoes, chopped

1 handful of pitted black olives, roughly chopped

60g cheese *(such as feta, Cheddar, mozzarella or Parmesan)*, torn or grated

Pasta salads are delicious with fresh raw vegetables, but I think they hold up better with roasted veg, and I love the flavour that roasting brings. It also stops your salad from getting soggy – no soggy salads here! Use any type of pasta you like; I prefer smaller shapes like orzo. This recipe works equally well for a packed lunch or a party, and you can roll over any leftovers for enjoying later.

Preheat the oven to 220°C/gas mark 9, then place the olive oil in a large roasting tin and pop in the oven to heat up.

Add the peppers, courgettes and red onion to the roasting tray and toss in the hot oil with the oregano, garlic and some salt and pepper. Spread out evenly in the roasting tray and roast in the oven for about 25 minutes, tossing halfway through, until the veg are tender and going golden at the edges.

Meanwhile, mix the dressing ingredients together in a large serving bowl and season with salt and pepper.

In strongly simmering salted water, cook the orzo until al dente (according to the packet instructions) – usually 7–9 minutes.

Drain the orzo and add to the serving bowl – it's good if there's still a little starchy water clinging to the pasta as this helps makes a luscious dressing – then toss to combine.

As soon as the roast veg are ready, add them straight to the serving bowl along with any juices from the roasting tray, then toss again, season with salt and pepper to taste and leave to cool, although this is really delicious at any temperature – I often have one portion warm and then eat another portion cold the next day.

Once cooled, or whenever you're ready to eat, toss with the herbs, tomatoes, olives and cheese and divide between lunchboxes, or serve up at room temperature to a party of friends or at a picnic.

variations

Stir in a big spoonful of pesto (page 123), or a little spoonful of harissa.

For a plant-based option, swap the cheese for a handful of toasted pine nuts or your favourite nuts or seeds.

herbaceous tomato salad with honey halloumi and chimichurri drizzle

feeds 4 as a side ———— 10 minutes

400g ripe cherry tomatoes, halved

250g halloumi, patted dry and
   sliced into 12 pieces

1 tsp runny honey or maple syrup

chimichurri drizzle

1 handful of fresh coriander

1 handful of fresh parsley

1 handful of fresh chives or spring
   onions, roughly chopped

1 big garlic clove, finely chopped

2 tbsp apple cider vinegar or
   lemon or lime juice

4 tbsp extra-virgin olive oil

1 tsp dried oregano or thyme,
plus extra to serve

A pinch of chilli flakes or a little
   chopped fresh chilli

Sea salt and black pepper

I love how the refreshing salad complements the salty fried halloumi, but it would be delicious on its own too. The drizzle is inspired by chimichurri – a delicious herby dressing from Argentina and Uruguay. If you've got a handful of watercress, rocket, radish leaves or carrot tops to use up, finely chop and add them too for an extra green boost, and save on food waste as a bonus. To make this more substantial, add beans, lentils or roasted sweet potato.

———————————————————————————

First, make the chimichurri drizzle. Rough chop the leaves of the coriander and parsley and finely chop the stalks, then add to a bowl and mix with all the other ingredients, seasoning with salt and pepper to taste. Alternatively, roughly blitz the chimichurri ingredients in a food processor.

Add the tomatoes to a serving platter and mix with half of the chimichurri drizzle. Serve the rest on the side or save for another salad.

Pop a large frying pan on a medium-high heat and fry the halloumi for 1 minute or so on each side until golden. Transfer to a serving plate and drizzle over the honey or maple syrup, along with an extra sprinkling of dried oregano or thyme. Enjoy straight away with the tomato salad while the halloumi is still warm.

greek-style buckwheat, feta and olive salad

feeds 2 as a main or 4 as a side ——— 25 minutes

125g buckwheat *(the unroasted kind)*, rinsed and drained
2 tbsp olive oil
1 handful of fresh dill
1 handful of fresh mint or parsley
1 handful of cherry tomatoes, halved
⅓ cucumber, sliced into half moons or chopped
1 red pepper, deseeded and chopped
½ small red onion, finely sliced
2 handfuls of black *(Kalamata)* olives, pitted
100g feta, roughly chopped
Sea salt and black pepper

oregano-garlic dressing
Juice of 1 lemon or 2 tbsp red wine vinegar
4 tbsp extra-virgin olive oil
1 tsp dried oregano, plus extra to serve
¼ tsp Dijon mustard
½ garlic clove, finely chopped
A pinch of ground cumin and cinnamon *(optional)*

This is inspired by the universally adored Greek salad, with buckwheat for extra heartiness. Buckwheat isn't exciting on its own, but is fantastic at soaking up dressings and sauces. Give it a try instead of rice, quinoa or grains like spelt or farro. Make this salad 'cold-day friendly' by roasting the red pepper and cherry tomatoes for 30 minutes, which is super delicious and makes for a more warming dish. For extra pizzazz, add some chopped dates, pistachios or pomegranate seeds to the salad and sprinkle ½ teaspoon of dried mint over the feta.

———————————————————————

Cook the buckwheat in a medium pan on a medium heat for 3 minutes to evaporate off the excess water, then add the olive oil and fry for 5 minutes, stirring every so often until it smells toasty. Add 250ml of water and a little pinch of salt and simmer for 10 minutes with the lid on until tender but not soft.

Drain and rinse the buckwheat under cold water to cool it down quickly. Shake the sieve to get rid of any excess water and then transfer to a medium wide bowl (that you can serve from).

Mix together all the dressing ingredients in a small bowl, or shake in a clean screw-top jar, seasoning with salt and pepper to taste, then pour over the buckwheat in the bowl.

Roughly chop the dill and the mint or parsley leaves and finely chop the stalks of the dill and parsley (if using), then add to the serving bowl with the rest of the salad ingredients except the feta, and toss everything together. Finish by scattering over the feta and sprinkling extra dried oregano over the top to serve.

warm potato and watercress salad with asparagus

feeds 4 as a side ———— 20 minutes

500g new potatoes, scrubbed

200g asparagus spears, ends
snapped off *(see tip)*

2 tbsp capers

2 tbsp chopped cornichons

2 spring onions or 1 small handful
of fresh chives, chopped

1 handful of fresh parsley or dill,
finely chopped

2 handfuls of watercress or
pea shoots

Sea salt and black pepper

2 soft-boiled eggs, halved,
to serve *(optional)*

dressing

Juice of 1 lemon and a little
grated zest

2 tbsp extra-virgin olive oil

½ tsp wholegrain or Dijon
mustard

2 tbsp natural yoghurt or
crème fraîche

My absolute favourite potato salad. This gets rave reviews around my way during the spring and summer months. It's just what I'm after in warmer weather – special enough for a party and crowd-pleasing at a picnic. When asparagus isn't in season, I use green beans, which need twice as long to cook, or tender-stem broccoli. When you can't get new potatoes, any waxy potatoes will work, just roughly chop them after they are cooked.

Bring a medium pan of salted water to the boil and drop in the potatoes. Simmer on a medium heat for about 15 minutes, depending on the size and type, until tender to the point of a knife. Add the asparagus spears to cook for the final 3 minutes, and then drain.

While the potatoes are cooking, mix all the dressing ingredients together in a serving platter, then add the capers, cornichons, spring onions or chives and the parsley/dill and season with salt and pepper to taste.

Add the drained potatoes to the serving platter with the asparagus and watercress or pea shoots. If using large potatoes, roughly chop them. Toss everything together in the dressing and finish with an extra sprinkling of black pepper. Top with the eggs, if using.

tip

Snap the bottom inch off the end of each asparagus spear and save for making stock or soup.

feel good

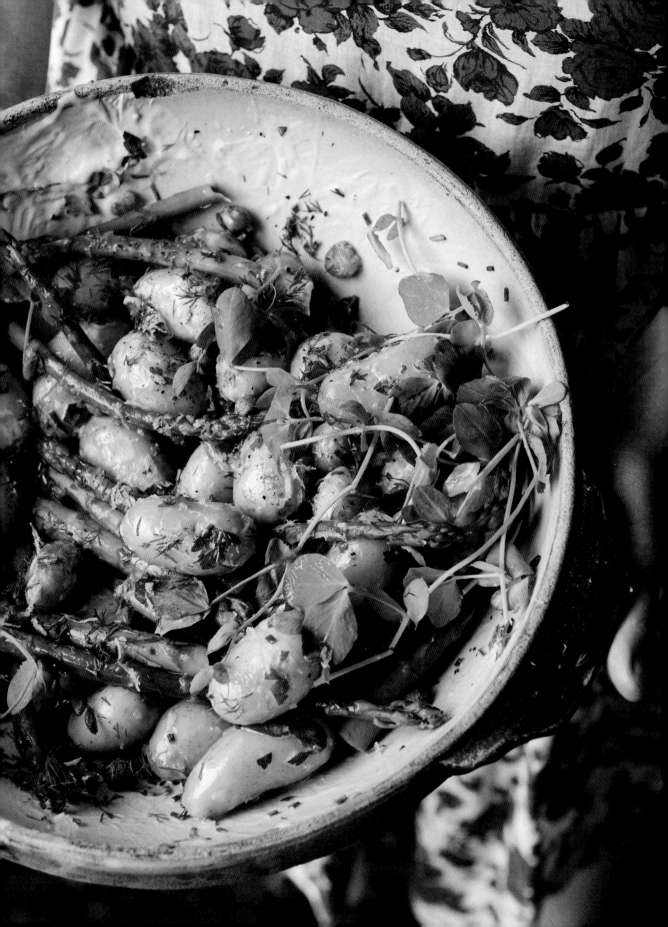

quick leeky beans

feeds 2 as a main ———— 20 minutes

2 tbsp ghee or extra-virgin olive oil
1 medium leek, finely sliced *(see tip)*
2 garlic cloves, finely chopped
400g tin of white beans *(such as
  butter beans)*, drained and rinsed
Juice and grated zest of ¼ lemon
1 handful of artichoke hearts
  (from a jar), roughly chopped
Sea salt and black pepper

to serve
1 small handful of fresh parsley
  or basil, roughly chopped
1 handful of grated Parmesan,
  Pecorino or Cheddar
A drizzle of extra-virgin olive oil

A humble tin of cooked beans is speedily transformed into a very delicious hearty dish that I eat as often for brunch as for dinner. When leeks are in season, I get so many in my weekly veg box and this is one of my go-to ways to enjoy them. You've probably got most of these ingredients in your cupboard or fridge already. The addition of artichokes and a sprinkling of cheese makes this extra special.

In a medium frying pan, heat the ghee and fry the leek on a low–medium heat for 6 minutes, stirring from time to time and adding the garlic to cook during the final 2 minutes.

Add the beans, a good pinch of salt and pepper and fry for 3 minutes, adding a splash of water if needed.

Stir in the artichokes and lemon juice and zest and cook for a final minute, then taste for seasoning and scatter with the fresh herbs and the grated cheese and drizzle over a little olive oil.

variation

Turn this into 'braised leek soup' by adding 300ml veg stock.

tip

Save the darker green leaves of the leeks to use in casseroles, stocks or soups – wash the leeks really well, as they pick up a lot of dirt.

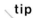

feel good

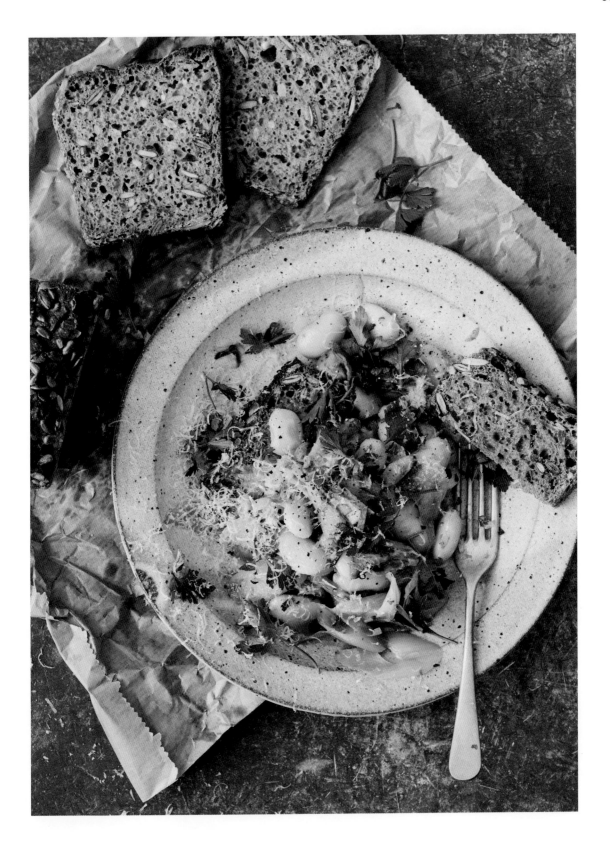

lunchbox heroes and satisfying salads

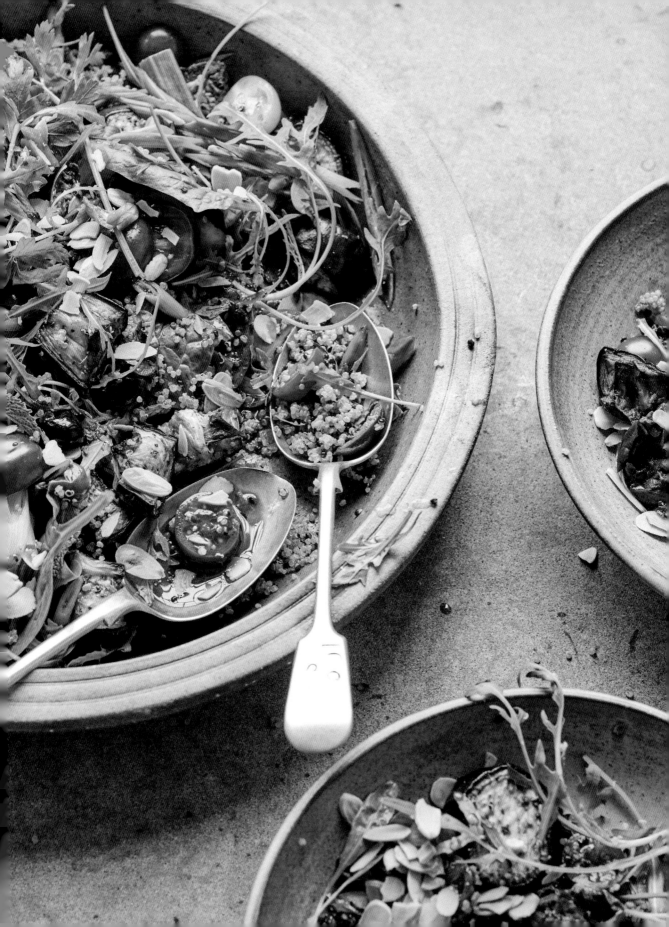

aubergine and tomato salad
with harissa-honey dressing

feeds 4 as a main ———— 30 minutes

2 tbsp ghee or olive oil

3 small aubergines *(about 800g)*, cut into chunks

1 tsp dried thyme or oregano

2 handfuls of whole or flaked almonds

200g quinoa or buckwheat, rinsed

400ml veg stock

2 handfuls of ripe cherry tomatoes, halved or quartered

4 spring onions, finely chopped

2 handfuls of pitted olives, halved

2 big handfuls of rocket or mixed leaves, roughly chopped

2 big mixed handfuls of fresh basil or parsley, roughly chopped

Sea salt and black pepper

harissa-honey dressing

2 tsp *(rose)* harissa paste *(or to taste, depending on the brand)*

Juice of 1 lemon and a little grated zest

2 tsp runny honey or maple syrup

4 tbsp extra virgin-olive oil

This salad is lovely both at room temperature, while the aubergine and quinoa are still warm, or cold. I prefer smaller aubergines to larger ones as I think they taste better. This is also good with basil or coriander if you have some in the garden, and I often swap spring onions for chives in the summer when they grow and grow and grow. I love serving this with feta sprinkled over at the end or shavings of a hard cheese like Pecorino or Parmesan.

Preheat the oven to fan 220°C/gas mark 9, then place the ghee in a large roasting tray and pop in the oven to heat up.

Carefully toss the aubergine chunks in the hot ghee with the dried herbs and a good pinch of salt and pepper, then spread out in the roasting tray in a single layer and roast for 15 minutes. Toss well in the tray and roast for another 10–15 minutes until the aubergine is completely tender and getting nicely golden at the edges.

Meanwhile, toast the almonds in a saucepan on a medium heat for a minute or so on each side until fragrant, then roughly chop, if using whole almonds, and set aside.

Pop the pan back on the heat and cook the quinoa or buckwheat in the veg stock according to the packet instructions, with a lid on the pan, until tender (usually about 15 minutes for quinoa and 12 minutes for buckwheat). Leave to stand off the heat for a few more minutes, then fluff with a fork and transfer to a biggish, wide serving platter.

Make the dressing by mixing all the dressing ingredients together and shaking in a clean screw-top jar or whisking with a fork in a bowl. Pour over the quinoa, toss, then set aside for 5 minutes to cool.

Add the tomatoes, spring onions, olives, rocket and half the herbs to the serving platter and toss everything together well. Scatter over the toasted almonds along with the rest of the herbs.

10-minute carrot salad
with cumin dressing

feeds 4 as a side ———— 10 minutes

3 large carrots *(about 500g)*
1 handful of raisins, roughly
  chopped
1 handful of fresh parsley,
  coriander or mint, chopped
1 handful of flaked or whole
  almonds

cumin dressing
1 tsp ground cumin
3 tbsp extra-virgin olive oil
Juice of 1 small lemon and a little
  grated zest
1 tsp Dijon or wholegrain mustard
1 tsp maple syrup or runny honey
A little pinch of chilli flakes
Sea salt and black pepper

It's always handy to have a vegetable side dish that can go with everything, isn't it? A great salad to have on a picnic or for a packed lunch with some cooked lentils. This is delicious as it is, or add a tin of chickpeas or beans to make it instantly more filling and satisfying – just make sure to double the amount of dressing. Store leftovers in the fridge for a day or so and use them to brighten up wraps or as a topping for a black bean soup.

Mix the dressing ingredients together in a serving bowl, seasoning with salt and pepper to taste.

Scrub the carrots rather than peeling them, then use a box grater to roughly grate them. Add the grated carrots to the bowl, along with the raisins and half the herbs, toss everything in the dressing and season with salt and pepper to taste. Pop the salad into the fridge to chill for 10 minutes or longer, if you have the time.

Meanwhile, put a frying pan on the hob and toast the almonds with a pinch of salt on a medium heat for 3–4 minutes, shaking halfway through, until lightly golden all over. If using whole almonds, tip onto a chopping board and roughly chop.

Serve the salad with the nuts and remaining herbs on top.

fried halloumi slaw

feeds 4 as a side ———— 15 minutes

½ small red cabbage
1 fennel bulb or 2 celery sticks
1 large carrot, scrubbed
1 ripe *(but not too soft)* pear or
  apple, unpeeled
1 handful of fresh herbs *(such as
  parsley, coriander or mint leaves)*
1 big handful of nuts and seeds
  (such as pecans and sunflower seeds)
250g halloumi, patted dry and
  chopped into chunks
1 tsp Aleppo chilli flakes or ½ tsp
  regular chilli flakes
1 tsp dried oregano or thyme

honey-vinegar dressing
2 tbsp apple cider vinegar
2 tsp wholegrain or Djion mustard
4 tbsp extra-virgin olive oil
2 tsp runny honey, plus 1 tsp
  to serve
Sea salt and black pepper

Quick, crunchy, fresh and colourful, this such a good side all summer long and for barbecue feasts. To make this heartier to eat as a main, toss in some roasted sweet potatoes or cooked quinoa, noodles, rice or lentils, or stuff it in a wrap. I need no excuse whatsoever to fry up some halloumi with a drizzle of honey, but halloumi is best hot, of course, so if you want to take this on a picnic, swap the halloumi for some crumbled feta.

Start by mixing the dressing ingredients together with a fork in a medium serving platter, seasoning with salt and pepper to taste.

Use a sharp knife or a vegetable peeler to shred your cabbage into nice thin slices, then add it to the platter and toss in the dressing.

Finely slice the fennel/celery, carrot and pear/apple, then add them to the bowl, along with the fresh herbs. Peel the carrot into ribbons with the vegetable peeler, if you like.

Heat up a large frying pan and toast your nuts and seeds on a medium heat for 3–4 minutes until golden, then tip them onto your chopping board and very roughly chop any big nuts.

Pop the pan back on a medium heat and fry the halloumi pieces, undisturbed, for about 1½ minutes on each side until golden brown – space out the halloumi to make sure they fry rather than steam. In the last 30 seconds of cooking, sprinkle over the chilli flakes and dried herbs. Tip the halloumi onto your slaw and drizzle a final teaspoon of honey on the halloumi. Serve straight away while the halloumi is still warm. Leftover slaw will last 2 days.

pictured on page 181

charred corn and avocado salad

feeds 4 as a side ——— 30 minutes

2 large corn on the cob, shucked
  (about 500g)
1 red pepper, deseeded and diced
100g feta, very roughly crumbled
1 handful of fresh coriander,
  stems finely chopped and leaves
  roughly chopped
3 tbsp extra-virgin olive oil
1 small ripe avocado, peeled and
  roughly chopped
Spicy Lime-pickled Red Onion
  (page 246)
Sea salt and black pepper

One of my favourite picnic and barbecue salads, this always goes down a storm. Fresh corn on the cob is ideal but if it is out of season, add some frozen or tinned sweetcorn to a hot frying pan and cook for 4–5 minutes until you get some charred bits. Serve this with tortilla chips or as part of a feast with **Fish Finger Tacos** (page 211).

Either preheat the grill to the highest setting and cook the corn for 20 minutes, turning halfway through, or grill on the barbecue or in a griddle pan on the hob for 5 minutes on each side until deeply golden brown in places.

Place the remaining ingredients, except the avocado and pickled red onions, in a serving bowl, add a pinch of salt and pepper and mix together well.

Once the corn is cool enough to handle, slice the kernels off each 'ear' and gently mix into the bowl. I like to slice off big chunks, if I can, but any way it comes off is good! If you like, for ease, slice the ears in half first so you have four ears, and then slice off the kernels.

When you're ready to serve, add the avocado, pour over the lime juice from the pickled red onions and gently toss. Scatter over the pickled onion to finish.

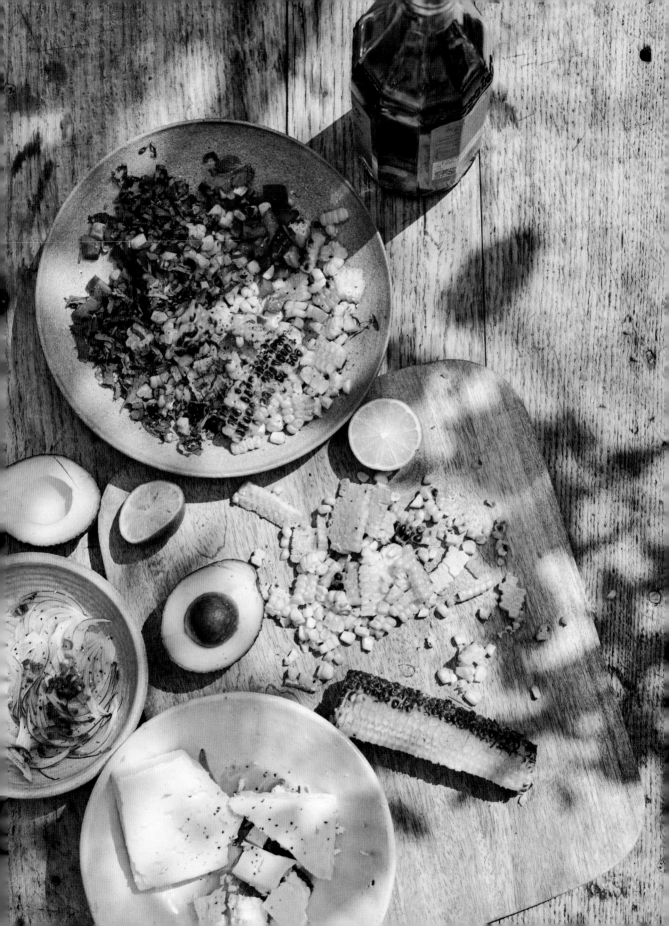

sweet potato salad
with peanut-lime sauce

feeds 4 ———— 40 minutes

2 tbsp coconut oil or ghee
2 sweet potatoes, scrubbed
200g extra-firm tofu
1 handful of new potatoes
1 tsp curry powder
3 eggs
200g green beans
1 large pepper, deseeded
  and sliced
½ cucumber, sliced
2 handfuls of torn lettuce
Sea salt and black pepper

peanut-lime sauce
50g smooth peanut butter
2 tbsp tamari or soy sauce
2 tbsp lime juice
1 tbsp maple syrup or coconut
  sugar
1 fresh chilli, deseeded and
  chopped, or ½ tsp chilli flakes
1 garlic clove, finely chopped
4 tbsp coconut milk (optional)

optional extras
Toasted coconut flakes or
  crushed peanuts
1 handful of chopped fresh
  coriander or spring onions
Lime wedges

Inspired by *gado gado* (meaning 'mix mix'), one of my favourite Indonesian dishes, this makes a satisfying veg-packed supper or easy party-pleasing salad. The peanut-lime sauce is definitely one to have up your sleeve and can be made with any nut butter. This is traditionally made with boiled potatoes and fried tofu, but I love this way of roasting half the salad and keeping the other half of the salad raw for a beautiful contrast.

Preheat the oven to fan 220°C/gas mark 9, then divide the coconut oil between two large baking trays and place in the oven to heat up.

Meanwhile, slice the sweet potatoes (without peeling them) into 1cm-thick rounds. Pat the tofu dry in a clean tea towel and chop into bite-sized pieces. Make sure everything is dry so it doesn't spit in the hot oil.

Take out both trays from the oven, then carefully tip the sweet potatoes and whole new potatoes into one tray and toss in the hot oil with a good pinch of salt and pepper. Add the tofu and curry powder to the second tray and toss in the hot oil (using tongs or a couple of forks). Arrange everything in each tray so that it's spread out as much as possible and in a single layer, then roast for 15 minutes.

Meanwhile, boil the eggs for 8 minutes in a pan of salted water.

feel good

Make the sauce by mixing all the ingredients together in a small bowl, adding a pinch of salt and 2 tablespoons of hot water, continuing to add more water as needed until the sauce is thick but pourable. Taste for seasoning and adjust if needed (you might not need to add extra sea salt because of the tamari/soy), so that you've got a lip-smackingly delicious balance of salty, tangy, creamy and a little bit sweet and spicy.

Once the 15 minutes of roasting time is up, take out the baking trays and divide the green beans (top them first but don't bother tailing) between the two trays and toss with the other ingredients, then spread out in a single layer on each tray and roast for another 10–15 minutes. Swap the trays around so that whichever was on top goes to the middle, and vice versa, and cook until the veg are tender and the tofu is going golden at the edges.

Arrange the raw veg on a big serving platter with the peeled and quartered eggs, then add the roasted veg and tofu once they are ready and drizzle over a few big spoonfuls of the sauce. Top with any of the optional extras and serve with the rest of the sauce on the side for everyone to help themselves to more.

pictured overleaf

variation

I love to eat seasonally as much as possible. In spring, enjoy this with broccoli, asparagus, radishes and lots of spring onions. In the winter, roast some cauliflower or Brussels sprouts and pumpkin, and use shredded red cabbage and carrots instead of the peppers and tomatoes.

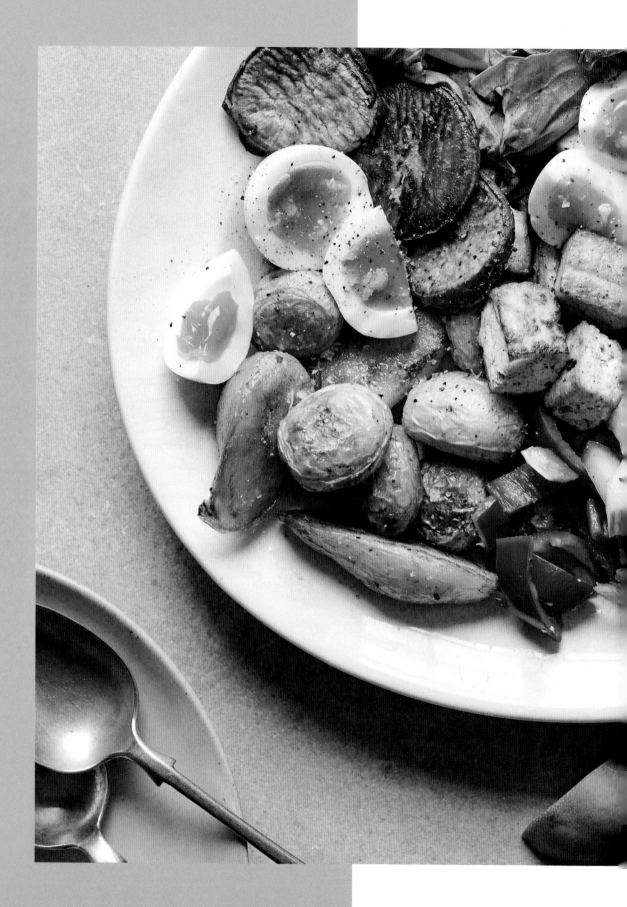

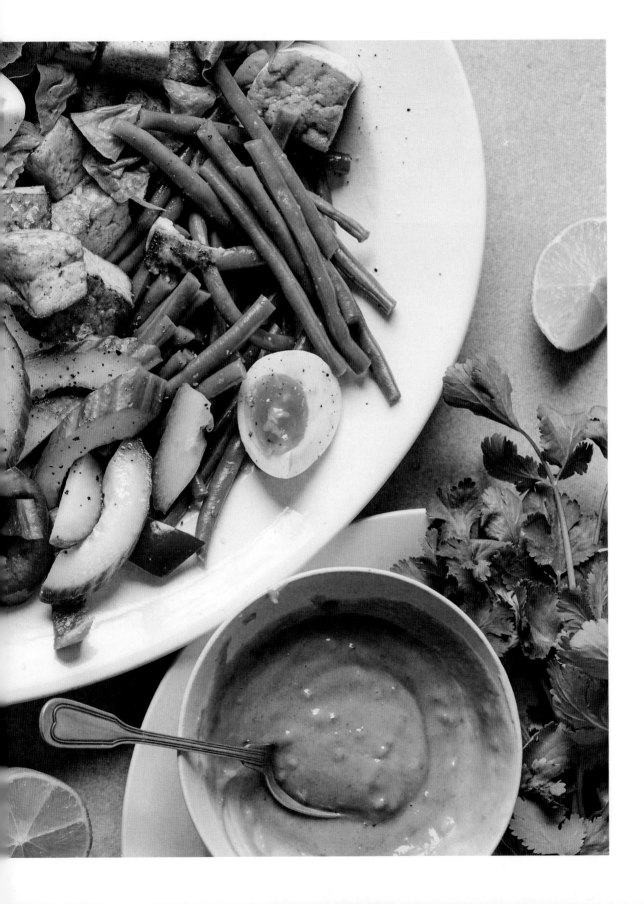

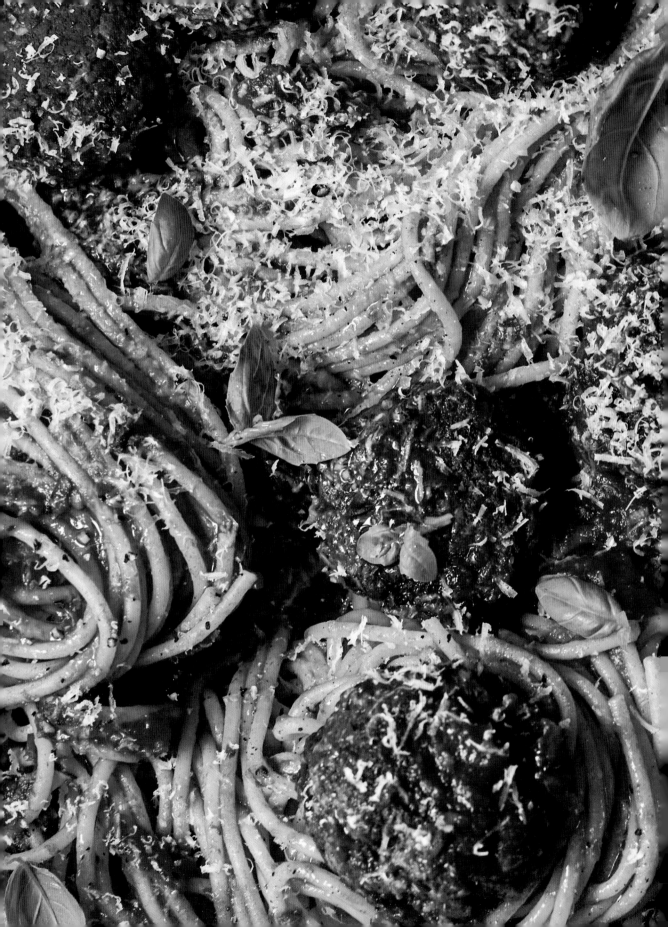

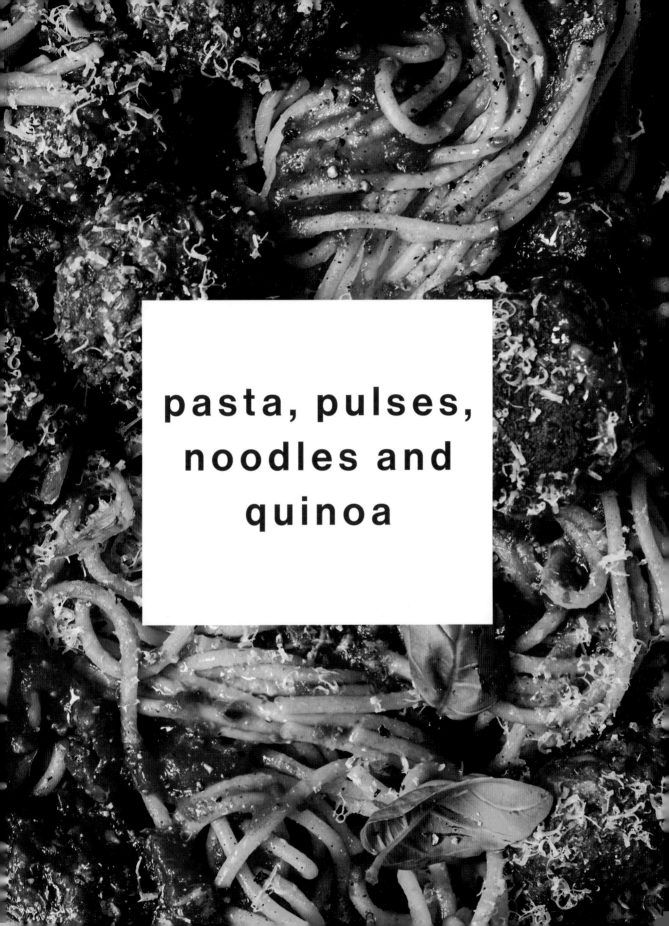

pasta, pulses, noodles and quinoa

/ ideal for flexible cooking /

These recipes are inspired by those trusty tins and packets of good old dried goods in our kitchen cupboards – ready to go, convenient, great for making meals go further and ideal for flexible cooking. Recipe-wise, you'll find lots of comforting family-friendly favourites in this chapter, but with some veg-packed twists and flavour-boosting additions.

Just as I always recommend variety when it comes to veg, my motto is to change it up with your store-cupboard staples. A gentle weekly (or even monthly) meal plan really helps here. In the past I found it all too easy to get stuck in the rut of putting the same ingredients into my shopping basket every week, but it's always best for your gut to eat a diverse range of foods, plus it keeps things interesting, especially when other members of the family get to choose what's for dinner! A few years ago I challenged myself to eat as many different sorts of pulses as I could, including chickpeas and all types of bean, as well as different types of noodles. My favourite are buckwheat (soba) noodles and pasta shapes made from quinoa, chickpeas or lentils.

The key store-cupboard ingredient in many of the recipes here can be exchanged for something else. **Sesame-Peanut-Lime Noodles** (page 111)? Swap the noodles for leftover fried rice next time. **Spaghetti and Veg Balls in Tomato Sauce** (page 120)? Enjoy the veggie mushroom balls spooned over chickpea mash or **Farinata** (page 218). **Creamy Mushroom and Spinach Pasta** (page 128)? Try the delicious mushroom and spinach mixture stirred through some fluffy cooked quinoa or with buckwheat on the side. Don't miss out on making the **Veg-packed Mac 'n' Cheese** (pages 114–16) and if, like me, you regularly make a noodle stir-fry, you'll now be wanting to top your bowls with those gorgeous **Omelette Ribbons** that I just can't get enough of (page 132). They make a simple weeknight stir-fry really special.

In other chapters, look out for:

- **Any Bean, Any Lentil Chilli** (page 66)
- **Cosy Coconut Lentils with Kachumber** (page 64)
- **Lunchbox Orzo Pasta Salad** (page 89)
- **One-pan Oregano Chicken and Chickpeas** (page 192)
- **Quick Leeky Beans** (page 94)
- **Roasted White Beans with Caesar-style Tahini Dressing** (page 76)
- **Kedgeree-style Smoked Mackerel** (page 26)

roasted broccoli and tofu with sesame-peanut-lime noodles

feeds 2 ——— 30 minutes

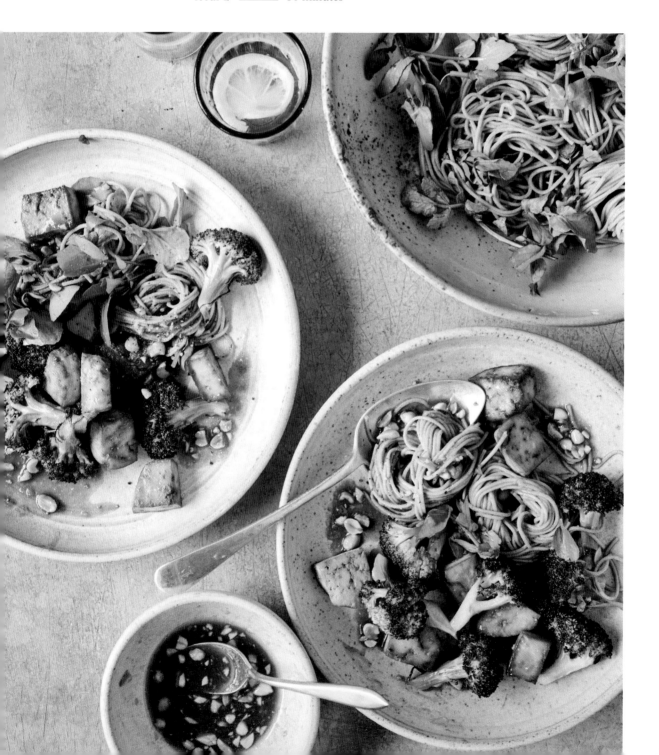

280g extra-firm tofu, drained

1 tbsp tamari or soy sauce

2 tsp maple syrup

1 large head of broccoli

1 tbsp coconut oil

2 bundles of dried soba noodles or spaghetti

2 handfuls of watercress or baby spinach, roughly chopped

1 lime, quartered, to serve

sesame-peanut-lime dressing

1 handful of peanuts or cashews

1 large garlic clove, finely chopped or grated

2.5cm fresh ginger, finely grated

1 tbsp tamari or soy saue

2 tsp maple syrup

1 tsp white or brown miso paste

2 tsp toasted sesame oil

3 tbsp extra-virgin olive oil

A pinch of chilli flakes or a dash of chilli sauce

Juice of 1 lime

Veg-packed and full of flavour, this makes a perfect weekday supper. If you don't have miso, not to worry: add a touch more tamari, but consider getting yourself a small jar of miso as it adds an incredible depth of flavour to Japanese- and Korean-inspired dishes and to lentils and mushrooms in shepherd's pie or ragù. Use any type of miso here. White miso tends to be sweeter, so you if you're using it, you might want to add a touch less maple syrup.

Preheat the oven to fan 220°C/gas mark 9. While it's heating up, scatter the nuts for the dressing on a large roasting tray and toast for 5–10 minutes, keeping an eye on them, until they're nicely golden. Tip out onto a chopping board, then roughly chop and set aside.

Meanwhile, chop the tofu into 1.5cm cubes, pat dry (in a clean tea towel) and mix with the tamari and maple syrup in a small bowl.

Chop the broccoli into equal-sized florets, then trim the stem of any knobbly bits and slice into pieces. The stem is denser than the florets so needs to be chopped smaller to cook in the same time.

Let the coconut oil melt briefly in the hot roasting tray, then tip the tofu onto the tray and toss in the oil. Space out in the tray and roast for 10 minutes. After 10 minutes, toss the broccoli with the tofu on the tray, space out again and roast for another 8–10 minutes until the tofu is golden and the broccoli is tender.

Mix the dressing ingredients together in the bowl that held the tofu and add the chopped nuts.

Cook the noodles according to the packet instructions, reserving half a mug of the cooking water. Take the noodle pan off the heat and tip the noodles back in, then add the chopped watercress or spinach and a dash of cooking water and mix together.

By now the broccoli will be tender and golden-edged, like the tofu, so combine everything together (in the roasting tray, if you like, to save washing-up) and add most of the dressing, plus another splash of noodle water if needed. Serve with the rest of the dressing and the lime wedges on the side.

crab and courgette spaghetti

feeds 4 ——— 15 minutes

400g dried spaghetti

3 tbsp butter or olive oil, plus
  extra to finish *(optional)*

4 spring onions, finely sliced

3 big garlic cloves, finely chopped

1 fresh red chilli, deseeded if
  you prefer and finely sliced,
  or a good pinch of chilli flakes,
  plus extra to serve *(optional)*

2 medium courgettes, roughly
  grated *(400g)*

200g British crab meat *(150g
  white and 50g brown meat)*

1 big handful of fresh parsley,
  finely chopped

2½ tbsp lemon juice and ½ tsp
  grated zest

Sea salt and black pepper

1 handful of grated Parmesan,
  to serve *(optional)*

This reminds me of both Italy and Scilly (not Sicily!) – the beautiful Isles of Scilly, 27 miles off the coast of Cornwall, where I've eaten the tastiest seafood of my life. This dish is speedy but special. When I have friends coming over, it is a fail-safe meal that looks and tastes impressive but is ready in a flash, so I can relax and spend time with my loved ones. Good-quality crab meat is expensive but a little goes a long way. I find this combination of three parts white crab meat to one part brown goes down a treat.

Bring a large pan of salted water to the boil, with a lid on for speed, then add the spaghetti and cook according to the packet instructions – I cook it for just under a minute less than the specified time. Drain the spaghetti, reserving a mugful of the starchy cooking water.

Once the spaghetti is in the pot, heat up the butter in a large, deep-sided frying pan, add the spring onions, garlic and chilli and stir-fry on a medium heat for 2 minutes, letting the garlic soften but not brown. Add the grated courgette and a generous pinch of salt and pepper, then turn up the heat, mix everything together well and fry for another 4 minutes, stirring regularly, until the courgette liquid evaporates.

Take off the heat and stir in the flaked crab meat, parsley and lemon juice and zest.

Quickly add the spaghetti to the crab pan, adding around half a mug of the reserved pasta cooking water and gently tossing as you go, so you get a beautiful glossy sheen. Add more of the pasta cooking water if needed, and you could add an extra drizzle of olive oil or knob of butter at this stage. Taste for seasoning and serve straight away with some extra chilli or black pepper and the grated Parmesan, if using (I am pro seafood and cheese!).

variation

Swap the crab for 4 handfuls of chopped artichoke hearts and olives and omit the Parmesan for a delicious veggie alternative.

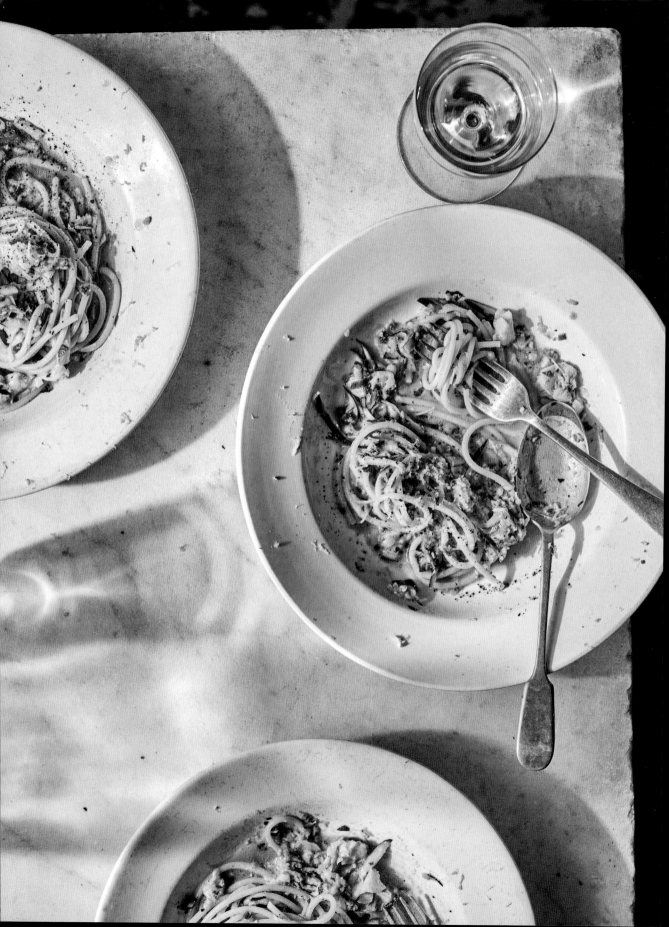

veg-packed mac 'n' cheese

feeds 4 ———— 1 hour *(hands-on time 20 minutes)*

350–400g dried pasta shapes
  (I love conchiglie)
500g mix of cauliflower
  and broccoli
40g butter
2 garlic cloves, finely chopped
40g buckwheat flour *(or any flour)*
A little pinch each of smoked
  paprika and ground nutmeg
700ml milk
1 generous tsp mustard *(any kind)*
200g mature Cheddar, roughly
  grated
50g Gruyère or Parmesan *(or
  more Cheddar)*, roughly grated
200g cherry tomatoes, halved
Sea salt and black pepper
A little chopped fresh jalapeño
  or a dash of chilli oil, to serve
  (optional)

Who doesn't adore mac 'n' cheese? I really love loading it with vegetables and this is the combo I make the most – cauliflower and broccoli, plus tomatoes for extra zip. Go for full-flavoured cheese here, such as mature Cheddar; otherwise you end up using twice the amount to get the right flavour hit. I like the variety in flavour of using two different cheeses, but just go for one, if you prefer. And serve with a big green salad to balance the richness with freshness. Perfect comfort food.

Preheat the oven to fan 220°C/gas mark 9 and bring a large saucepan of salted water to the boil. Cook the pasta for 2 minutes less than the packet instructions, as it will cook further in the oven. If the instructions say 10 minutes, for instance, you need to cook it for only 8 minutes.

Meanwhile, chop your florets into small bite-sized pieces and cut the stalks into 5mm chunks. I leave the broccoli florets a bit bigger than the cauliflower pieces as broccoli cooks a touch more quickly.

When the pasta has one more minute left to go, drop in the cauliflower and broccoli florets to cook with the pasta for a minute.

Drain the pasta and veg in a colander, reserving a generous mugful of the starchy pasta cooking water. Briefly run some cold water over the mixture in the colander to cool it, then tip into a large baking dish (about 30cm × 20cm).

In a medium saucepan (use the one you just used to cook the pasta), melt the butter on a medium heat, stir in the garlic and gently fry for 2–3 minutes. Add the flour and whisk pretty much continuously for around 3 minutes while you sprinkle in the paprika, nutmeg and some salt and pepper.

continued overleaf

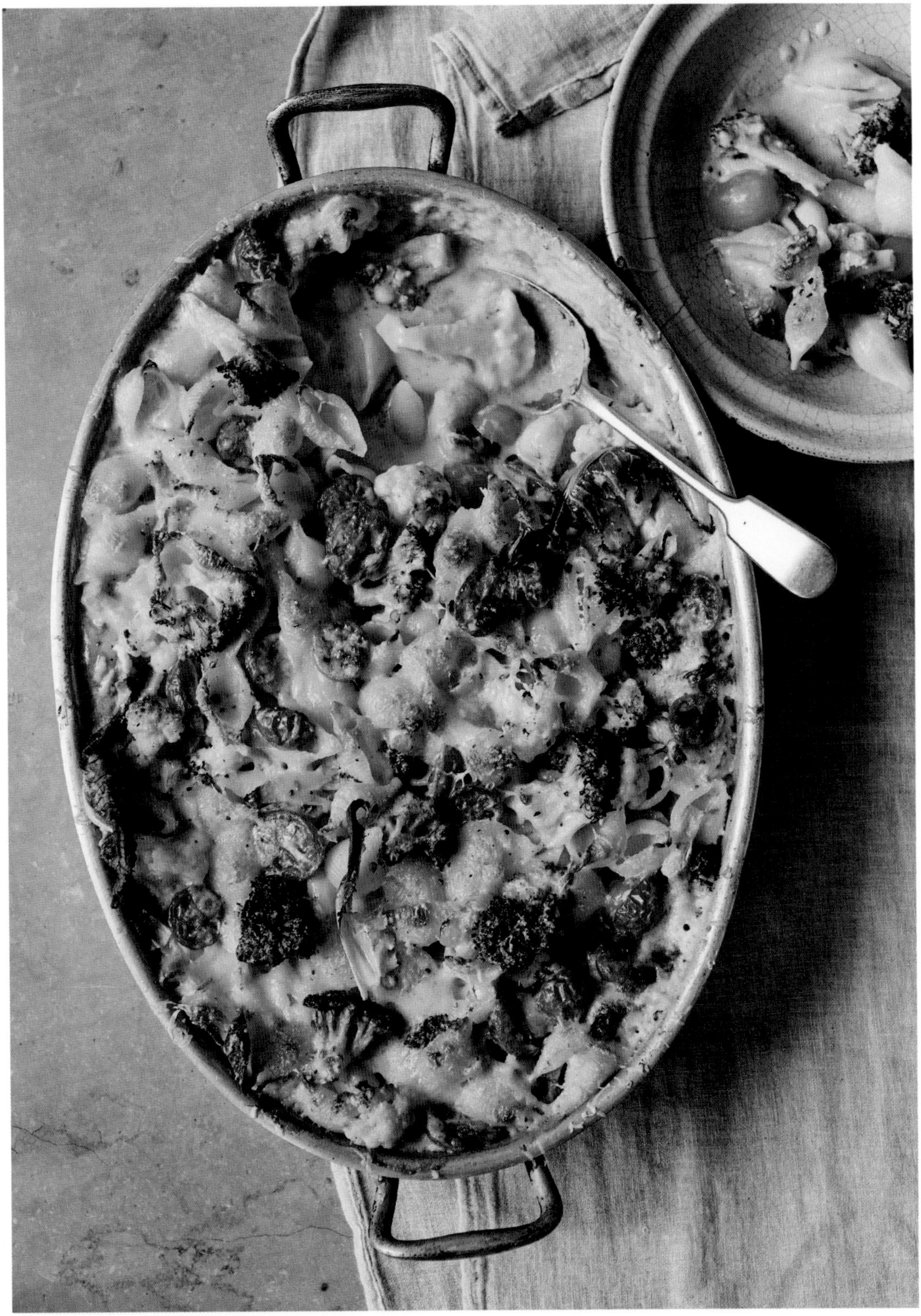

pasta, pulses, noodles and quinoa

After the 3 minutes, start adding the milk, about a fifth at a time and whisking constantly until all the milk has been combined and the mixture is smooth. Take the pan off the heat and stir in the mustard and three-quarters of the grated cheese, stirring until smooth and seasoning with salt and pepper to taste. Add the reserved pasta cooking water a little at a time until you reach your desired consistency (I like my mac 'n' cheese quite saucy so I add half a mug to begin and then add more as needed once stirred through).

Pour the cheese sauce into the dish, then toss gently to combine. At this point, if you think the pasta mixture needs more liquid, gently stir in some more of the cooking water. Spread everything out in the dish – there's no need to smooth it all out as you'll get lovely golden bits if pieces of veg and pasta poke out. Sprinkle over the last of the cheese, top with the halved cherry tomatoes and bake for 25 minutes. If, by the end of the cooking time, the top layer hasn't turned golden brown, either crank up the heat to maximum or turn on the grill to high, and cook for another 5 minutes or so, keeping an eye on it to make sure it doesn't burn.

Remove the mac 'n' cheese from the oven and, if you can bear to wait, allow the dish to sit for 10 minutes or so before diving in.

tip

To get ahead, cool the pasta and veg straight after cooking, cool the cheese sauce and make it sauce thinner with pasta cooking water before combining with the cooled pasta and veg. This stops the pasta and veg from cooking any further. Store, covered, in the fridge for up to 2 days.

green pasta ~ three ways

feeds 4 ——— 20 minutes

Creamy and smooth, this lovely green sauce is naturally plant-based as it's made with cashews. There are lots of greens in here and the peas work really well to add extra creaminess and natural sweetness to balance the darker greens. For more sensitive taste buds you could add more peas and less kale/cavolo nero, or use baby spinach in place of the kale/cavolo nero, adding it at the same time as the peas. You can change it up in so many different ways – I've given the basic method followed by three delicious variations.

100g kale or cavolo nero,
  roughly chopped
100g frozen peas
350–400g dried pasta of
  your choice
1–2 garlic cloves *(to taste)*, peeled
60g cashews
8 tbsp extra-virgin olive oil
Sea salt and black pepper

basic method

Bring a large saucepan of water to the boil with a big pinch of salt. Add the kale or cavolo nero and cook for 1½ minutes. Tip in the peas and cook for another 30 seconds, then scoop out all the veg with a sieve and transfer to a blender or food processor. Add the pasta to the same pan of water and cook until al dente (according to the packet instructions).

Add the rest of the ingredients to the blender or food processor, with a splash of the pasta cooking water, then season with salt and pepper and blend until smooth. If the sauce seems too thick, add a splash more of the pasta water. Taste for seasoning: you can always add more garlic or some chilli if you like. Once the pasta is cooked, drain and toss straight away in the pan with the green sauce. Serve with any of the extras you like from one of the three variations on the next page.

continued overleaf

tips

Save the kale stems for another dish, such as finely chopped and added to stir-fries, egg-fried rice or a frittata.

Reserve a few extra cashews for toasting and adding on top of the finished dish, if you like.

pasta, pulses, noodles and quinoa

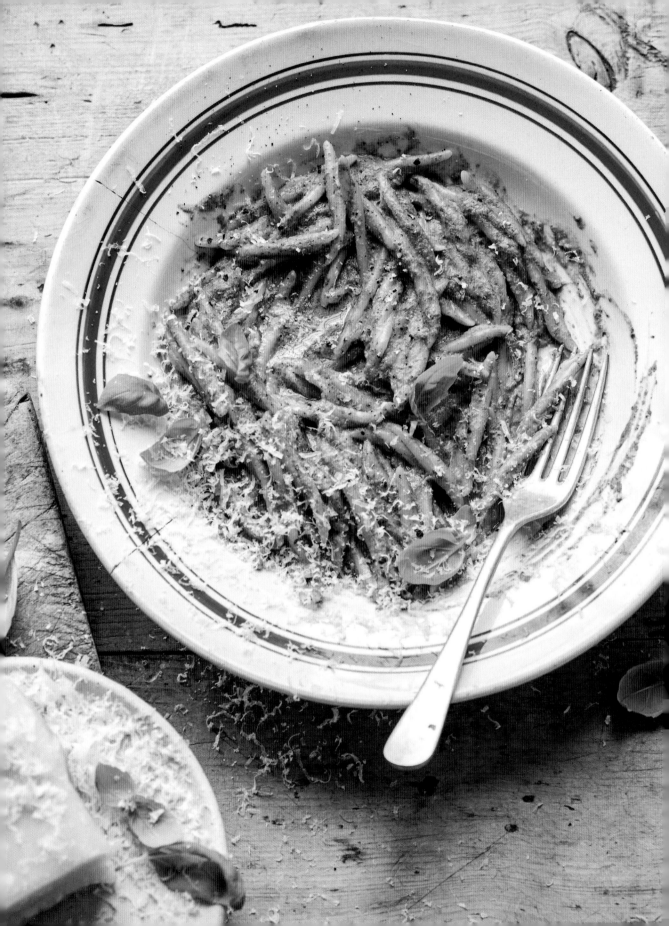

1/ feta, oregano and pistachio

100g kale or cavolo nero, roughly chopped
100g frozen peas
350–400g dried pasta of your choice
1–2 garlic cloves *(to taste)*, peeled
60g cashews
8 tbsp extra-virgin olive oil
1 tsp dried oregano, plus extra to serve
A pinch of chilli flakes
½ tsp grated lemon zest, plus extra to serve
Sea salt and black pepper

to serve (per bowl)
1 handful of crumbled feta
1 handful of pistachios

optional extras
1 handful of chopped olives
A squeeze of lemon juice

Follow the basic method, adding the oregano, chilli flakes and lemon zest to the blender or food processor with the other ingredients for the green sauce. Serve with the feta and pistachios – toasted for 3–4 minutes in a dry pan then chopped – and any optional extras scattered on top.

3/ parmesan and basil

100g kale or cavolo nero, roughly chopped
100g frozen peas
350–400g dried pasta of your choice
1–2 garlic cloves *(to taste)*, peeled
60g cashews
8 tbsp extra-virgin olive oil
Sea salt and black pepper

to serve (per bowl)
1 handful of grated Parmesan
1 handful of fresh basil leaves

optional extras
1 handful of chopped toasted pine nuts
1 handful of chopped olives
A squeeze of lemon juice

Follow the basic method and serve with the Parmesan and basil leaves and optional extras scattered on top.

2/ ginger and spicy sesame noodles

This variation is a bit different. I've added a few of my favourite Asian flavours to the green sauce – ginger, sesame and tamari. Use whatever noodles you like – buckwheat (soba) would work well here. I love this freshly made and hot, as it is here, but it's equally delicious cold.

100g kale or cavolo nero, roughly chopped
100g frozen peas
350–400g dried noodles of your choice
1–2 garlic cloves *(to taste)*, peeled
60g cashews
6 tbsp extra-virgin olive oil
2cm or more fresh ginger *(to taste)*, roughly chopped
2 tsp–1 tbsp toasted sesame oil *(to taste)*
Juice of 1 lime
Sea salt and black pepper

optional extras
2 tsp tamari or soy sauce

to serve (per bowl)
A little chopped fresh green chilli or a pinch of chilli flakes
1 handful of black sesame seeds
1 handful of chopped fresh coriander, mint or basil

Follow the basic method, cooking the noodles until al dente according to the packet instructions (1 minute less than the stated time) and adding the ginger, toasted sesame oil, lime juice and tamari or soy sauce to the blender or food processor with the other ingredients for the green sauce. Serve straight away with the chilli, sesame seeds and fresh herbs scattered on top.

spaghetti and veg balls
in tomato sauce

feeds 4, makes 20 veg balls ——————— 1 hour

veg balls

1 medium onion

2 tbsp ghee or olive oil

250g mushrooms *(such as chestnut)*

2 large garlic cloves, peeled

½ tsp smoked paprika

1 tbsp mixed dried herbs *(or 1 tsp
each of dried oregano, thyme and
rosemary or basil)*

1 tbsp tomato purée

80g rolled oats

50g walnuts

2 tsp tamari or soy sauce

2 tbsp grated cheese

1 egg

400g tin of green or brown
lentils, drained and rinsed *(240g)*

Sea salt and black pepper

tomato and basil sauce

1 tbsp olive oil or butter

3 garlic cloves, finely chopped

Stalks from 1 handful of fresh
basil, finely chopped

1 tsp dried oregano or mixed herbs

1 tbsp tomato purée

2 x 400g tins chopped tomatoes

1 tsp maple syrup or sugar
(optional)

to serve

350–400g dried spaghetti

Fresh basil leaves

Extra grated cheese

Following the super-popular lentil mushroom 'bolognese' in my last book, **Eat Green**, I wanted to share this veggie ball version with you that also uses lentils and mushrooms to make an amazing alternative to minced meat. This is a more time- and pan-consuming recipe, but well worth it as it's ideal for batch cooking. You can use leftover veg balls in a wrap for lunch or use the tomato sauce as a base for Mediterranean-style vegetable bakes or lasagnes as well as for **Bean Bites** (page 63).

First make the veg balls. Finely chop the onion by hand or in the small bowl of a food processor. Heat up 1 tablespoon of the ghee in a large frying pan, add the chopped onion and fry on a medium heat for 5 minutes, stirring from time to time.

Meanwhile, finely chop the mushrooms (do this in the food processor too, if you like – no need to wash it out) and the garlic and add to the onions, stir well and add a good pinch of salt and pepper. Fry for about 5 minutes, stirring from time to time, until the mushroom liquid has evaporated and the mushrooms are going nicely golden.

Stir in the paprika and dried herbs and cook for a minute, then add the tomato purée and cook for another minute.

Add the oats and walnuts to the food processor (no need to wash it out) and briefly blitz, then add the tamari, cheese, egg and the cooked mushroom mixture, and briefly blitz again. Turn off the food processor, stir the mixture and scrape down the sides and then add the lentils and briefly blitz again until all the ingredients are combined but not smooth. The mixture should be dry and dough-like in texture. (If you feel it's too wet, blitz in a teaspoon of oats to soak up the liquid; if it's too dry, add 1–2 teaspoons of olive oil.)

continued overleaf

feel good

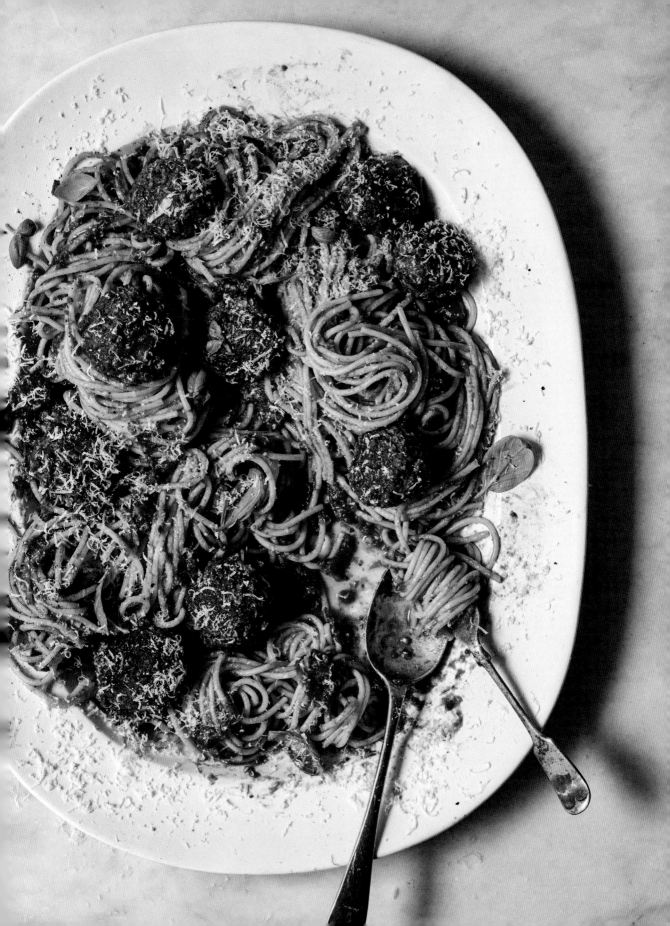

Roll into about 20 balls (roughly two bites each) using about 2 teaspoons of the mixture per ball. Pop them on a plate and place in the fridge to chill for 10 minutes to firm up. Meanwhile, preheat the oven to fan 190°C/gas mark 6½ and grease a large baking tray very well with the remaining ghee.

Next, make the tomato sauce. Heat up the olive oil in a medium saucepan, add the garlic, chopped basil stalks and dried herbs and fry on a medium heat for 3 minutes. Add all the remaining ingredients, pop a lid on the pan and cook on a medium simmer for about 10 minutes. Remove the lid and simmer for another 10 minutes to thicken and reduce. Season with salt and pepper to taste and add the optional 1 teaspoon of maple syrup or sugar if it needs it.

Place the veg balls on the greased baking tray and pop in the oven to bake for 20 minutes, until lightly browned. (See also tip.)

Meanwhile, bring a large pan of salted water to the boil, add the spaghetti and cook according to the packet instructions – I like to cook it for just under a minute less than the specified time. Drain the spaghetti, reserving a mugful of the starchy cooking water.

Stir the spaghetti into the pan of tomato sauce with a splash of the pasta cooking water, then serve up and top with the hot veg balls. Sprinkle over some grated cheese and basil leaves to finish.

variation

For a plant-based version, replace the cheese with 2 tablespoons of nutritional yeast. In place of the egg, use a 'flax egg' (page 245).

tip

If you'd rather skip the oven, place the veg balls back in the frying pan instead, and cook in the remaining ghee or oil on a low heat for 8 minutes per side, until lightly browned all over.

one-pan pesto chickpeas and broccoli

feeds 2 ——— 30 minutes

2 tbsp ghee or olive oil

1 head of broccoli

400g tin of chickpeas or beans, drained and rinsed

1 tsp dried thyme or oregano

A pinch of chilli flakes, smoked paprika, za'atar or harissa powder *(optional)*

pesto

2 tbsp nuts, such as cashews and almonds

1 large handful of fresh basil

1 handful of baby spinach, watercress or salad leaves

1 garlic clove

6 tbsp extra-virgin olive oil

2 tbsp lemon juice

Sea salt and black pepper

to serve

1 big handful of grated Parmesan, Cheddar or other hard cheese

2 handfuls of salad leaves

A firm favourite for a simple light supper, this is also delicious with cauliflower florets or with asparagus and green beans, which will need half the cooking time. Homemade pesto is super easy to make (and I like the fact that you can throw in a handful of spinach or salad leaves or herb stalks for extra flavour), but use shop-bought if you like. I recommend adding a squeeze of lemon if you do, to liven it up a little. To make the dish heartier, add cooked quinoa at the end.

Preheat the oven to fan 220°C/gas mark 9. Scatter the nuts on a large roasting tray and toast for a few minutes until lightly golden, then set aside. Return the tray to the oven with the ghee inside to melt.

Slice the broccoli into bite-sized florets and chop the stem pieces into roughly 1cm chunks. Pat the chickpeas or beans dry in a clean tea towel so they don't spit in the hot ghee.

Carefully tumble the broccoli and chickpeas into the melted ghee in the roasting tray and add the herbs and the spices (if using), plus a generous pinch of salt and pepper. Toss gently together and spread out in an single even layer – this helps the broccoli and chickpeas roast rather than steam. Place in the oven to roast for 15 minutes, then remove, toss, spread out again and roast for a final 10 minutes when the broccoli will be golden-edged and tender.

Meanwhile, make the pesto by adding the toasted nuts and seeds to a food processor with all the other pesto ingredients and blitzing everything together. Season with salt and pepper to taste.

Remove the broccoli and chickpeas from the oven and toss in 2–3 tablespoons of the pesto, scatter with the cheese and fresh leaves to serve.

sesame noodle salad with quick-pickled cucumber

feeds 2 ——— 20 minutes

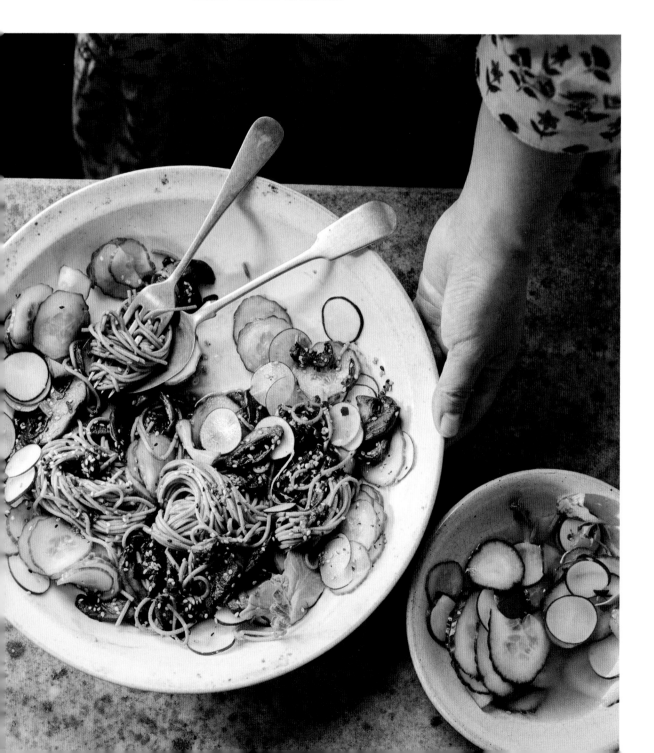

1 tbsp coconut oil or ghee

250g mushrooms, roughly sliced

1 fresh chilli, deseeded if
  you prefer, finely chopped,
  or a pinch of chilli flakes

3 tbsp mixed sesame seeds

2 bundles of dried soba noodles

Sea salt

quick-pickled cucumber

½ small cucumber

4 radishes

Juice of 1 lime

sesame dressing

1 garlic clove, finely chopped

1 tbsp rice vinegar or apple
  cider vinegar

1 tbsp tamari or soy sauce

2 tsp maple syrup

2 tsp toasted sesame oil

to serve

2 spring onions, finely sliced

1 handful of fresh coriander,
  finely chopped

Great for picnics and summer parties but simple enough for lunch at home or in a lunchbox to take to the park on a summer's day. The quick-pickled cucumber makes this extra interesting; quick-pickled carrot or just radish would be great too. Choose any mushrooms you like. My favourite is shiitake, but everyday chestnut mushrooms are less expensive and more widely available – a mix of shiitake and chestnut would be the ideal.

Finely slice the cucumber and radishes and pop into a small bowl with the lime juice and a pinch of salt. Stir well so the cucumber is fully coated in the lime juice and then set aside.

In a medium serving bowl, mix all the dressing ingredients together.

Heat up a large frying pan or wok and melt the coconut oil. Add the mushrooms and fry on a medium-high heat for about 5 minutes, tossing halfway through (it's best to not disturb them too much), until the mushrooms release their liquid and they start going golden at the edges. Add the chilli, sesame seeds and a pinch of salt, then stir-fry with the mushrooms for a final minute. Add to the serving bowl and mix with the dressing.

Bring a medium saucepan of water to the boil and cook the noodles (according to the packet instructions, typically around 4–5 minutes), then drain and immediately rinse in cold water. Shake off any excess water, then tip into the serving bowl and toss everything together well. You want to mix the noodles with the dressing straight away so that they don't stick together.

This salad is great warm or cold from the fridge. Just before serving, toss everything together with the spring onions and coriander and top with the quick-pickled cucumber.

store-cupboard sardine puttanesca with tagliatelle

feeds 4 ———— 30 minutes

2 tbsp ghee, butter or olive oil

1 large onion, finely chopped

4 garlic cloves, finely chopped

1 ½ tsp dried oregano or mixed herbs

A pinch of chilli flakes

2 medium carrots, scrubbed and finely grated

2 × 400g tins of chopped tomatoes

3 tbsp roughly chopped mixed olives and capers

1 handful of fresh basil or parsley, stalks finely chopped and leaves left whole

2 × 120g tins of good-quality sardines *(look for the ones in olive oil)*

A pinch of sugar *(optional)*

350–400g dried tagliatelle

Sea salt and black pepper

50g Parmesan or another hard cheese, finely grated, to serve

A quick, delicious pasta dish and a great way of enjoying more sardines. If your loved ones aren't sure about sardines, try one tin at first – that's what I did with my boyfriend. We've progressed to two tins because he loves it! I recommend grating carrots into tomato sauces; it takes seconds, adds sweetness and they disintegrate. You've already got the grater out for the cheese (yes – I am pro cheese with fish!), so why not get an extra portion of veg too?

Heat a medium saucepan and melt the ghee, then add the onion and a pinch of salt and fry on a medium heat, stirring every now and then, for about 6 minutes. Add the garlic, dried herbs and chilli flakes and cook for another minute.

Tip the grated carrots into the pan and fry for 3–4 more minutes. Add the tomatoes, then swill out the tins (to capture all the tomato juice) with about another 100ml of water and pour into the pan. Turn up the heat and simmer strongly for 10 minutes to reduce the liquid before adding the olives, capers and chopped basil or parsley stalks.

Once the sauce has thickened and reduced, add most of the sardines to warm through – they will break up in the sauce as you stir them. I like to save one fillet per person to serve on top. Taste for seasoning, adding a touch of sugar if you think it needs it, though the carrots should add sweetness to the sauce.

Meanwhile, get your tagliatelle on to cook in a saucepan of boiling salted water. Cook according to the packet instructions until al dente. Drain the tagliatelle, reserving a mugful of the starchy cooking water. Tip the tagliatelle into the pot of sauce and stir to combine, adding a few splashes of the reserved water if you want to loosen the sauce, then take off the heat.

Serve up each bowl with the saved sardine fillet on top, then scatter over the herbs and let everyone help themselves to cheese.

feel good

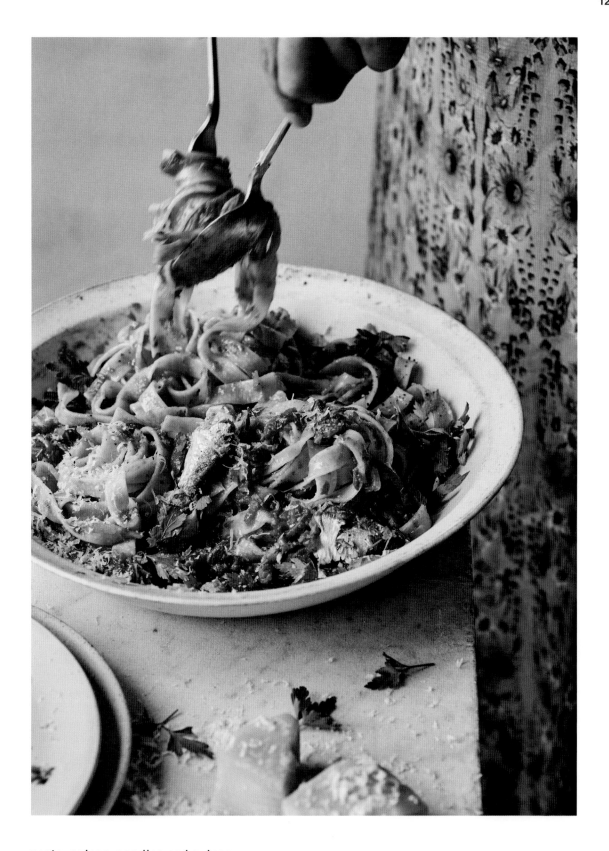

pasta, pulses, noodles and quinoa

creamy mushroom and spinach pasta

feeds 2 ———— 25 minutes

1 tbsp butter or olive oil

1 small onion, finely chopped

300g mushrooms *(such as chestnut or portobello)*, roughly chopped

½ tsp smoked paprika

½ tsp dried thyme

2 garlic cloves, finely chopped

200ml veg stock

1½ tbsp flour *(such as plain or chickpea/gram)*

1 tsp mustard *(any type)*

3 tbsp grated Parmesan cheese, plus extra shavings to serve

200ml milk

100g baby spinach

2 tbsp thick natural yoghurt or crème fraîche

175g dried pasta of your choice

Sea salt and black pepper

1 handful of fresh parsley or chives, finely chopped, to serve

Inspired by beef stroganoff, this is a veggie recipe with options to make it entirely plant-based (see variation). I like both versions, tossed through pasta, as it is here, or noodles or on top of mashed potatoes or rice. It would also be delicious with crusty bread or **Farinata** (page 218). For optional oomph, add 1 teaspoon of tamari or Worcestershire sauce (vegan, if needed) for an instant intense boost of flavour.

In a deep-sided medium frying pan, heat the butter and fry the onion on a low heat for 8 minutes, stirring regularly.

Add the mushrooms and a good pinch of salt and pepper, stir to combine with the onions and turn up the heat. Stir in the paprika, thyme and garlic and let the mushrooms fry away, releasing their liquid, for about 6 minutes or until they start to turn golden-edged. Stir regularly, adding a splash of the stock if needed.

Add the flour and fry for 30 seconds, stirring, then add the mustard and grated cheese. Pour in the stock and milk, then turn up the heat and let the mixture bubble away on a medium heat for 5 minutes. If you feel your sauce is getting too thick, let it cook with a lid on the pan to keep it 'saucy', which I prefer, but if you want your sauce thicker, simply cook without a lid.

Stir in the spinach and cook for another 2–4 minutes until the spinach has wilted, then stir through the yoghurt or crème fraîche and cook for a final minute until the sauce is hot and creamy.

Meanwhile, cook the pasta in a saucepan of boiling salted water (according to the packet instructions) until al dente. Drain the pasta, reserving a mugful of the starchy cooking water.

Season the sauce with salt and pepper to taste, then toss the pasta through the sauce – adding a splash or two of the reserved cooking water to loosen the sauce if needed – and sprinkle over the parsley or chives and shavings of cheese to finish.

variation

For a plant-based version, use plant-based milk and yoghurt/ crème fraîche and replace the cheese with 2 tablespoons of nutritional yeast.

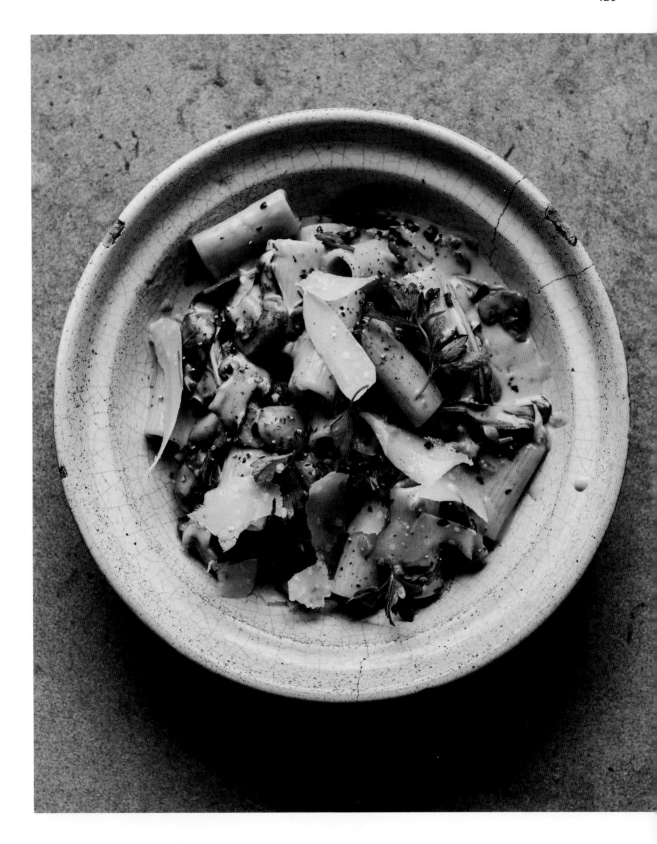

pasta, pulses, noodles and quinoa

zingy vietnamese-style noodles with fried sesame tofu

feeds 4 ——— 25 minutes

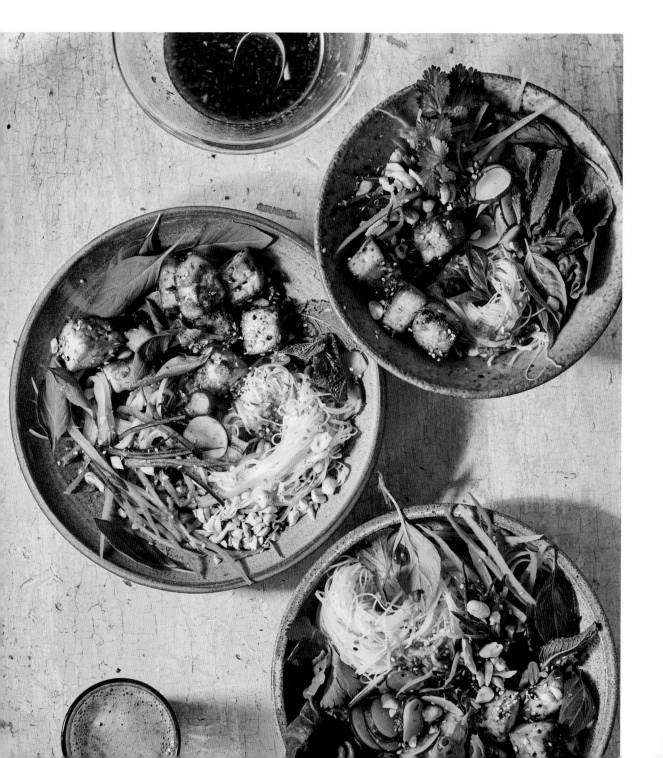

280g extra-firm tofu

2 tbsp coconut oil

1 tbsp maple syrup

2 tbsp mixed sesame seeds

dressing

Juice of 3 limes

2 tbsp maple syrup or
coconut sugar

2 tbsp fish sauce *(vegan if you prefer)*

2½ tbsp tamari or soy sauce

2 garlic cloves, finely chopped

1 Thai chilli, deseeded and finely
chopped, or 2 squirts of chilli
sauce *(or to taste)*

noodle salad

300g thin *(rice or mung bean)*
dried vermicelli

2 handfuls of mixed fresh herbs
*(such as coriander, basil and mint
– see tip)*

Leaves from 2 Little Gem lettuces

2 tbsp cashews or peanuts

2 carrots and ½ cucumber, sliced
into matchsticks

2 handfuls of finely sliced
radishes or cabbage

tip

Look out for Thai basil
and Vietnamese mint.

variation

Swap the tofu for 250g
mushrooms (my favourite are
shiitake), roughly chopped, and
fry in the same way as the tofu.

A must make! The sticky sesame tofu works beautifully in this dish, but you could swap it for mushrooms (see variation), prawns, shredded chicken or fish. This is one of my all-time favourite dressings. I also like to drizzle it on roasted cauliflower, baked squash and fried Brussels sprouts. I love thin rice vermicelli for speed, but cook up any type of noodles you like. This is also fantastic with leftover cooked rice or quinoa, and use vegan fish sauce to make this completely plant-based.

Mix the dressing ingredients in a small bowl or place in a clean screw-top jar and shake well.

Drain the tofu well. Chop into 2cm cubes, then pat dry in a clean tea towel. Pop into a bowl, stir in 2 tablespoons of the dressing and set aside to marinate for 10 minutes.

Meanwhile, place the dried vermicelli in a large, wide heatproof serving bowl, pour over some just-boiled water and leave for the length of time specified on the packet – usually around 5–8 minutes.

Keep the leaves of the fresh herbs whole and finely chop the stalks (discarding any mint stalks – or use in mint tea!) and tear the lettuce leaves.

Heat up a large frying pan, add the cashews or peanuts and toast on a medium heat for 2 minutes until lightly golden, then tip onto a chopping board and roughly chop.

Pop the pan back on the heat and melt the coconut oil. Using tongs, place the tofu pieces in the pan, spacing them out, and fry on a medium-high heat for 4–5 minutes, then turn over and cook for another 4 minutes. Try to leave them undisturbed as they fry so they go lightly golden and then, during the final minute of cooking, stir in the maple syrup and sesame seeds and remove from the heat.

Drain the noodles once they are tender (test one by eating it), wipe the bowl out with a clean tea towel and then pop the noodles back in the bowl, roughly snipping with scissors so they are easier to eat.

Drizzle over half of the dressing, add the herbs and veg and toss together in the bowl. Scatter over the tofu, then sprinkle the nuts on top to finish. Serve with extra dressing on the side so that everyone can add more if they like.

pasta, pulses, noodles and quinoa

simple stir-fried noodles
with omelette ribbons

feeds 2 ———— 20 minutes

2 bundles of dried noodles
  of your choice (*I like soba*)
2 tsp ghee or coconut oil
4 spring onions, white and green
  parts separated
2 garlic cloves, finely chopped
400g finely sliced mixed veg
  (*such as green beans, broccoli
  or cabbage*)
Chilli oil or spicy sauce, to serve

stir-fry sauce
3 tbsp tamari or soy sauce
2½ tsp toasted sesame oil
1 tsp maple syrup or coconut sugar

omelette ribbons
1 tsp ghee or coconut oil
2 eggs
1 tbsp black sesame seeds
  (*optional*)
Sea salt and black pepper

You're going to fall in love with these omelette ribbons. Make extra as they are delicious the next day added to salads. This is a family-friendly stir-fry, so the sauce isn't spicy, but you could serve it with a squeeze of chilli garlic sauce or **Red Miso Sauce** (page 72). I also like to add broccoli or cauliflower stems left over from other recipes, chopped up small, for the perfect speedy Monday night stir-fry.

Mix the sauce ingredients in a bowl or shake in a clean screw-top jar. Next, make the omelette. In a medium frying pan, heat up 1 teaspoon of ghee. Whisk the eggs with a good pinch of salt and pepper, then pour into the pan, tipping it from side to side so that it covers the bottom. Scatter over the sesame seeds, if using, and cook on a medium-high heat for about 2 minutes, then slide the omelette onto a chopping board or plate while you get on with everything else.

Bring a medium saucepan of salted water to the boil and cook your noodles (according to the packet instructions – usually around 4–5 minutes). As soon as they are just tender, drain them, reserving a mugful of the cooking water to use in the stir-fry sauce, and rinse with cold water to prevent sticking.

Meanwhile, pop the frying pan back on the heat and melt the rest of the ghee. Add the white parts of the spring onions and some of the green parts (saving the rest for garnishing at the end).

After a minute of stir-frying the spring onions, add the garlic and the mixed veg, then stir-fry on a high heat for about 5 minutes until just tender but still with some bite. Add the sauce, scraping the bottom of the pan as you stir it in, then add the noodles and toss together, adding a third to a half of the reserved noodle cooking water. Take off the heat, taste for seasoning and divide between bowls, topped with the reserved green parts of the spring onions.

Quickly finish by rolling the omelette up tightly into a sausage and slicing into ribbons before scattering over the top of each bowl. Serve with some chilli oil or spicy sauce on the side.

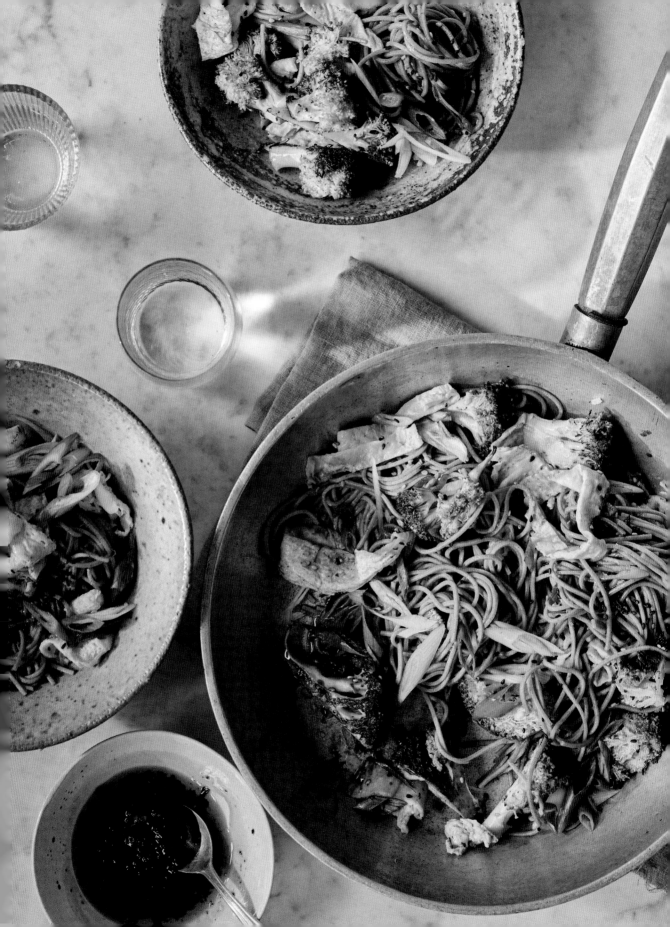

lemony spinach and feta quinoa

feeds 4 as a side ———— 30 minutes

3 tbsp butter or olive oil
1 medium onion, finely chopped
2 spring onions, finely chopped
2 large garlic cloves, finely chopped
1 tsp dried oregano, plus extra
  to serve
250g quinoa, rinsed well
800ml veg stock
200g baby spinach
1 handful of fresh dill or a mix of
  dill and parsley, chopped
Juice and grated zest of 1 lemon
150g feta
Sea salt and black pepper
A drizzle of extra-virgin olive oil,
  to serve

This zesty, cheerful, comforting dish of lemony and herby deliciousness is perfect for spooning straight from the bowl on a grey day. Inspired by the Greek spinach and rice dish *spanakorizo*, it is as delicious with quinoa as it is with the traditional rice, or try it with a mix of half rice and half quinoa. I love this as a simple quick main or as a side to fish or with roast tomatoes or peppers on top. Delicious hot or cold.

In a large, deep-sided frying pan, heat up the butter or olive oil, add the onion and fry on a medium heat for 5 minutes, stirring from time to time. Add the spring onions, garlic and oregano and fry for another minute with a pinch of salt and pepper.

Tip in the rinsed quinoa, turn up the heat, then stir to coat in the onion mixture and fry for 4 minutes to get a toasty flavour, stirring regularly.

Pour in the stock, then bring to a medium simmer and let the quinoa bubble away, adding a few splashes of water if you think it needs it, for about 13 minutes or until tender.

Add the spinach, most of the fresh herbs and half the lemon juice and zest, then let the spinach wilt for 2 minutes and gently mix it through. Season to taste with salt and pepper and the remaining lemon juice and zest, then crumble over the feta and sprinkle dried oregano over the feta. Finish with the last of the herbs and a drizzle of olive oil.

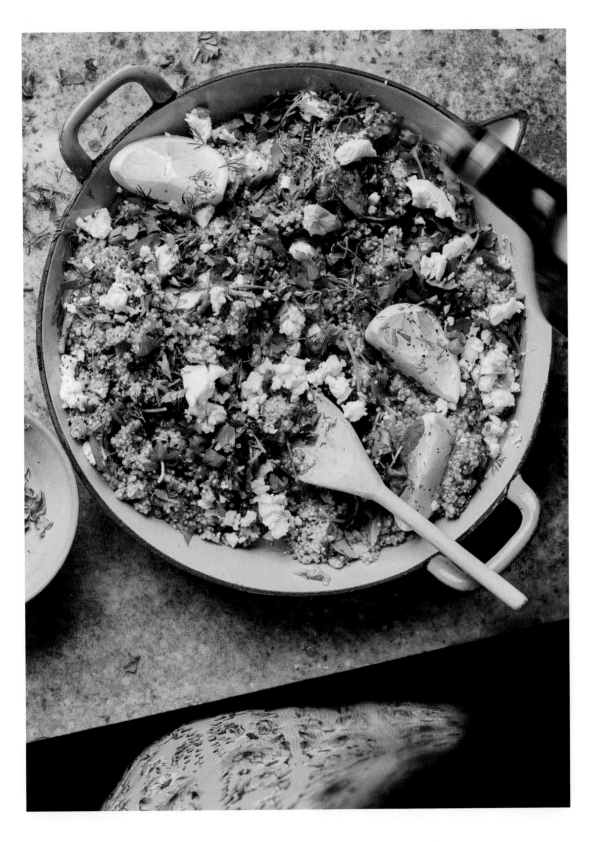

pasta, pulses, noodles and quinoa

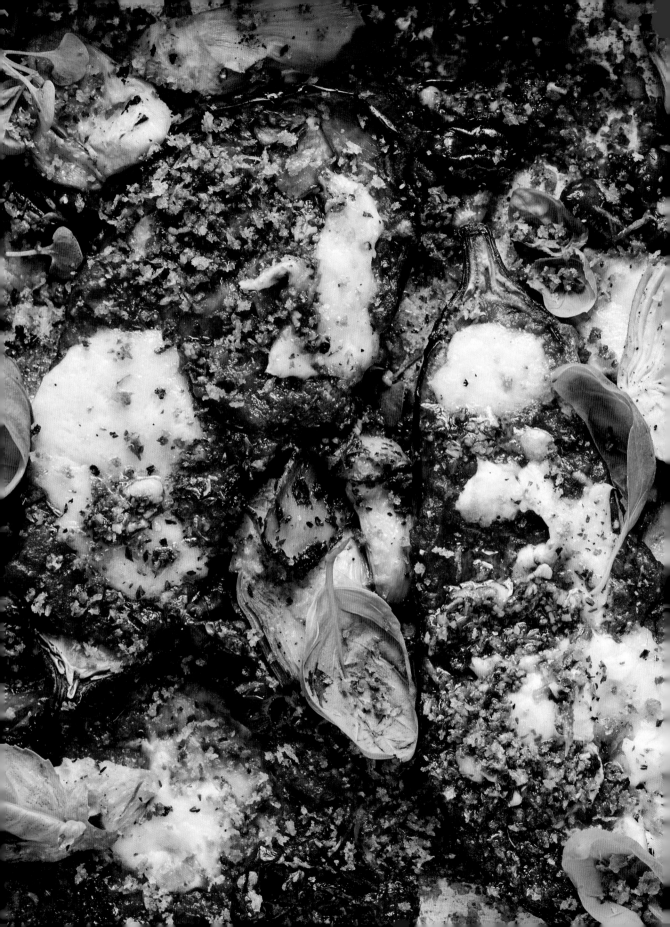

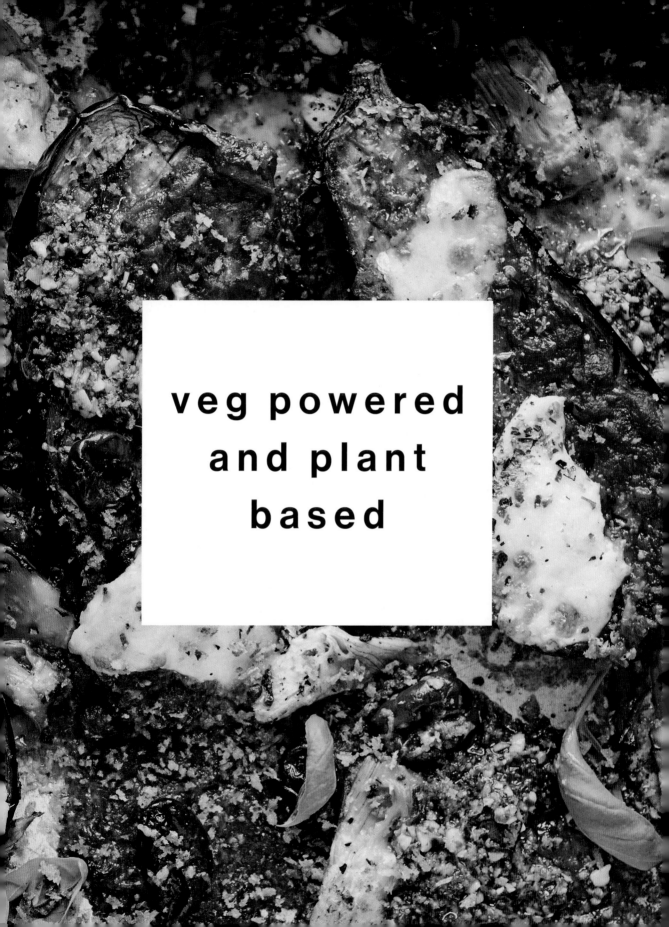

veg powered
and plant
based

/ vegetables are forever the star of the show /

Vegetables are forever the star of the show at mealtimes for me. I don't count the number of portions of veg I eat each day, but my plate is always full of them, in a vibrantly multicoloured mixture. You'll find the vegetables in this chapter are fresh for the most part, although I try to keep a freezer drawer filled with my favourites – frozen sweetcorn, peas, green beans, spinach and kale (dark leafy greens are top of my feel-good list and they're quick to cook too) – so I never run out of veg on busy weeknights.

Eating seasonally is one of the most delicious, sustainable and affordable ways to enjoy vegetables at their best, so let your shopping basket and plate be guided by nature and eat what's best according to the season. You can really taste the difference when something's grown and picked at the right time.

If it's not already a fully plant-based recipe, everything in this chapter can be tweaked to be vegan friendly; I've suggested alternatives along the way, but do also take a look at page 245 for vegan swaps and for taste tips and tricks, so you never need to compromise on flavour.

One of my favourite recipes in this chapter is the **Shiitake Mushroom Adobo** (page 154) – a vegetarian version of chicken adobo, the unofficial national dish of the Philippines that my mum (who comes from the capital Manila) cooked every week throughout my childhood in the suburbs of London. I also recommend the **Sweetcorn-Carrot Fritters** (page 146); they're a total hit with kids and make great party bites too. For a spiced twist on that nostalgic classic, eggs and beans, try the **One-pan Masala Beans with Eggs** (page 152). And I make the **shawarma-spiced sweet potatoes and cauliflower** (page 162) all the time. Enjoy it as part of a hearty vibrant salad or load it into a toasted wrap and top with the creamy **Tahini Yoghurt** (page 166). Don't forget the **pink pickled onion** (page 246) for a beautiful tangy flourish. For more delicious **homemade condiments**, **chutneys** and **vegetable pickles**, check out pages 246–7.

In other chapters, look out for:

- **Cosy Coconut Lentils with Kachumber** (page 64)
- **No-bake Chewy Nutty Bars** (page 227)
- **Roasted White Beans with Caesar-style Tahini Dressing** (page 76)
- **Scrambled Spiced Tofu** (page 18)
- **Three-Ingredient Chocolate Pots** (page 230)
- **Zingy Vietnamese-style Noodles with Fried Sesame Tofu** (page 131)

And many, many more!

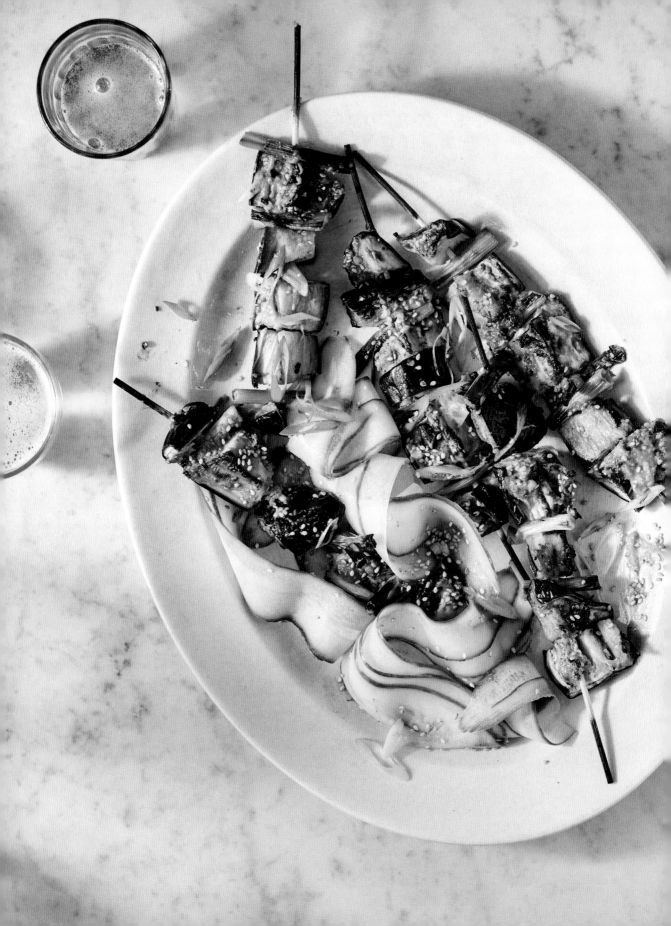

aubergine skewers
with cucumber ribbons

feeds 2 ———— 30 minutes

1 tbsp coconut oil or ghee
1 medium aubergine *(about 350g)*
6 spring onions, sliced into
   quarters

sauce
1 tsp finely grated fresh ginger
   (from a 2cm piece)
1 ½ tbsp white miso paste
2 tsp tamari or soy sauce
1 tbsp toasted sesame oil
1 tsp mirin, rice wine vinegar
   or apple cider vinegar
A pinch of black pepper or
   chilli flakes

to serve
½ cucumber
1 handful of sesame seeds
2 lime or lemon wedges

These delicious Japanese-inspired sesame miso skewers are cooked under the grill here, but you could cook them in a griddle pan on the hob or on a barbecue, if you prefer, and serve with quinoa or buckwheat. You could also pop the skewers in the oven at fan 220°C/gas mark 9 to cook for about 25 minutes, turning halfway through. Small young leeks are also a great alternative to spring onions, or just chop up a red onion and thread the chunks on.

———————————————————————

Preheat the grill to high, then place the coconut oil in a heatproof bowl and pop it under the grill for the oil to melt. Alternatively, melt the oil on the hob in a small saucepan.

Slice the aubergine in quarters lengthways and then roughly chop into 2.5cm pieces. Thread the aubergine pieces onto 4–6 skewers (depending on their length), alternating with the sliced spring onions (thread them on horizontally), then brush with the melted coconut oil. Place the skewers on a large baking tray and grill for 15 minutes, turning halfway, until tender and going golden at the edges. If the spring onion is starting to catch in the last few minutes, move the tray onto a lower rack so it is further away from the grill.

Meanwhile, mix all the sauce ingredients in the heatproof bowl, if using (no need to wash it out first), and taste for seasoning.

Take out the tray of skewers and close the grill door to keep in the heat. Brush the skewers all over with the sauce, then grill for another 3 minutes.

Use a vegetable peeler to peel the cucumber into ribbons. Pile these onto plates, along with any side you might be using, and then add the skewers once they are cooked. Scatter with the sesame seeds and serve with a wedge of lime or lemon to squeeze over the cucumber.

tip

I recommend investing in reusable skewers as they're so handy, but if you use bamboo ones, soak them in water for 15 minutes first or they will burn.

veg powered and plant based

cauliflower, cannellini and cherry tomato traybake

feeds 2 ——— 30 minutes

2 ½ tbsp coconut oil or ghee
½ cauliflower and a handful of
   cauliflower leaves *(600g total)*
400g tin of cannellini beans,
   drained and rinsed
250g cherry tomatoes
2 tsp curry powder
½ tsp cumin seeds or 1 tsp
   ground cumin
½ tsp fennel seeds
Sea salt and black pepper

coriander-lime yoghurt
100g Greek-style yoghurt
Juice of ½ lime and a little
   grated zest
½ small garlic clove
A little chopped fresh green
   chill or jalapeño
1 handful of fresh coriander,
   saving a few leaves to garnish

Enjoy this as it is or serve with your favourite side, such as quinoa, buckwheat or rice. Use any beans or chickpeas you like. I also love this served in a wrap (warm it in the oven for the last 5 minutes of the roasting time) or stuffed into a roasted sweet potato.

Preheat the oven to fan 220°C/gas mark 9, then place the coconut oil in a large roasting tray and pop it in the oven to heat up.

Meanwhile, prepare the cauliflower by cutting it into bite-sized florets and roughly chopping the leaves, keeping any smaller leaves whole. Dry the beans in a tea towel so they don't spit in the hot oil.

Add the cauliflower and beans to the heated tray, along with the tomatoes and spices, season with salt and pepper and carefully toss in the hot oil before spreading out in an even layer. Roast for about 15 minutes, then gently toss before roasting for another 10 minutes until the cauliflower and beans are golden at the edges and the tomatoes are collapsing. (If you are using very small cherry tomatoes, take them out sooner as they'll cook more quickly.)

Meanwhile, blitz the yoghurt ingredients together and season with salt. If you want to skip using a blender or food processor, then just grate or finely chop the garlic and finely chop the coriander, especially the stalks, though I personally love the creamy smoothness of the machine-blitzed yoghurt mixture as a contrast to the roast veg and beans.

Serve up in bowls, dolloping with the yoghurt to finish and topping with the reserved coriander leaves, or spread the yoghurt over the base of two plates and pile everything on top.

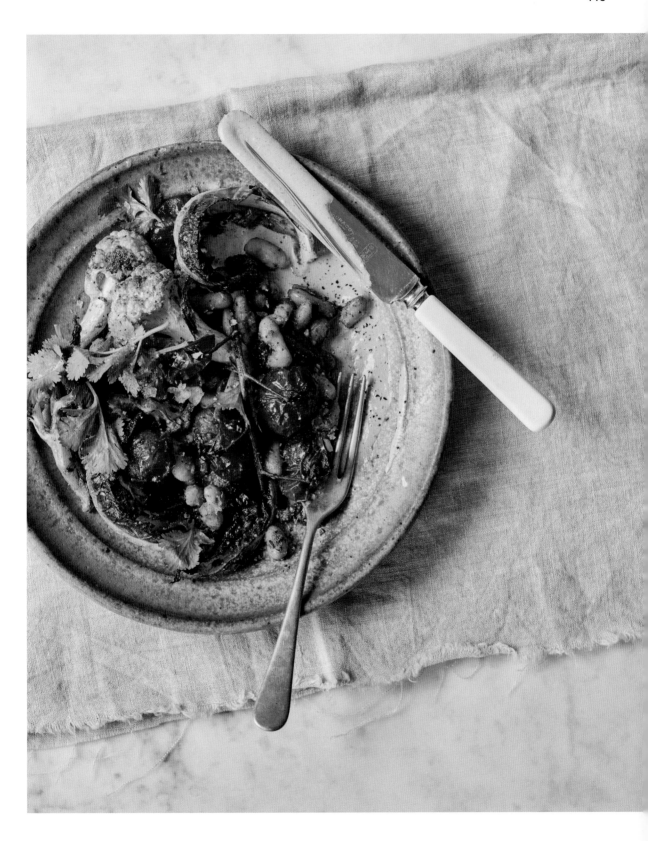

veg powered and plant based

halloumi veg traybake
with chilli-honey drizzle

feeds 3 ———— 40 minutes

3 tbsp ghee or olive oil
1 medium red onion
1 red, orange or yellow pepper
1 aubergine
1 courgette
4 garlic cloves, unpeeled
200g cherry tomatoes
1 ½ tsp dried oregano or thyme
400g tin of butterbeans or
  other beans/chickpeas, drained
  and rinsed
1 handful of pitted olives and
  sun-dried tomatoes *(optional)*
250g halloumi, roughly chopped
  into 16 cubes
Sea salt and pepper

chilli-honey drizzle

2 tsp runny honey *(or maple syrup)*
2 tbsp extra-virgin olive oil
A pinch each of chilli flakes and
  dried oregano

to serve

1 handful of roughly chopped
  fresh basil or parsley leaves
A few handfuls of rocket,
  watercress, lamb's lettuce or
  baby spinach *(optional)*

A fantastic one-tray dish to pack in loads of vibrantly coloured vegetables, this reminds me of Greek lunches and Mediterranean sunshine. The halloumi could be swapped for chunks of feta or some mozzarella balls, but halloumi is my definite favourite here. And do make the chilli-honey mix, which is really lovely drizzled on all cheese dishes – try it in a cheese toastie!

Preheat the oven to fan 220°C/gas mark 9, then place 2 tablespoons of the ghee in a large roasting tray and pop it in the oven to heat up.

Roughly chop the onion and all the other vegetables, except the cherry tomatoes, into bite-sized pieces, then remove the tray from the oven and tumble the veg, garlic and cherry tomatoes in the hot ghee, along with the oregano or thyme and a good pinch of salt and pepper. Toss together, then spread out in a single layer – to let them roast rather than steam – and roast for 15 minutes.

Remove the tray from the oven, add the beans and olives and sun-dried tomatoes, if using, toss together, then spread everything out again and roast for another 10 minutes.

Preheat the grill to high. Remove the garlic and toss everything else in the tray (for one final time!), then scatter the halloumi cubes on top and pop under the hot grill for 4–5 minutes or until the halloumi is golden brown, then turn over (tongs help here, or use a couple of forks) and grill for another few minutes on the other side.

Meanwhile, place the ingredients for the chilli-honey drizzle in a small bowl with a little pinch of salt and mix together well.

Serve up each plate, giving everyone a smooshed peeled garlic clove, then drizzle the chilli-honey mix over the halloumi and scatter over the herbs and any extra salad leaves, if you like, to finish.

feel good

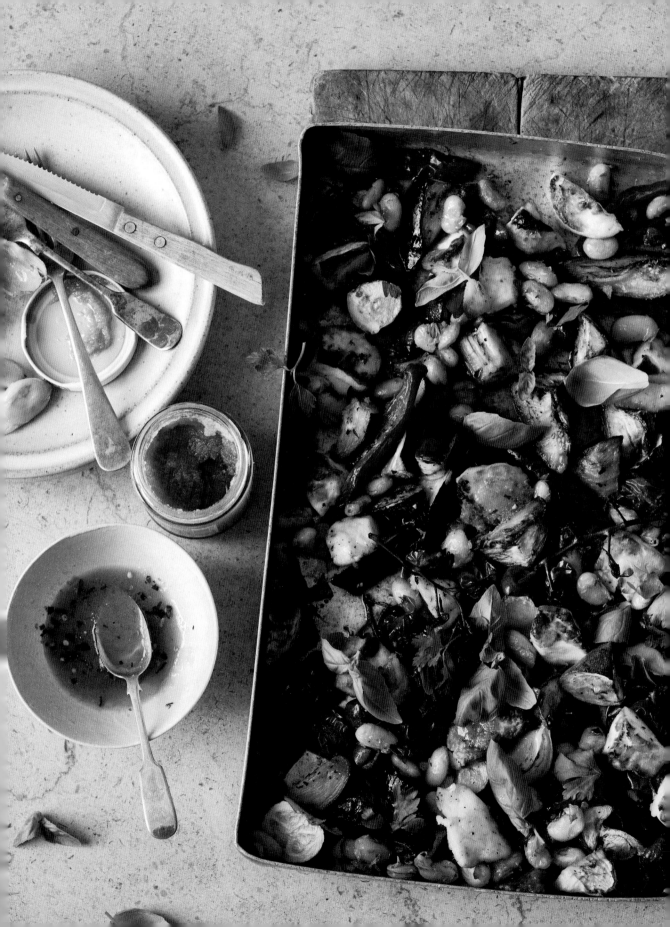

sweetcorn-carrot fritters with herby yoghurt and tomato salsa

serves 4 as a light main, makes 16 small fritters ———— 45 minutes

fritters

250g sweetcorn *(tinned and drained or frozen and defrosted)*

500g carrots, scrubbed and roughly grated

½ onion or 6 spring onions, finely chopped

1 large garlic clove, finely chopped

2 tsp curry powder

100g chickpea *(gram)* flour

¼ tsp baking powder

3 tbsp ghee or coconut oil, for frying

Sea salt and black pepper

herby yoghurt

6 tbsp Greek-style yoghurt or coconut yoghurt

3 tbsp chopped fresh mint leaves or coriander

1 small garlic clove, finely grated

tomato salsa

200g ripe tomatoes *(or cherry tomatoes)*, diced

2 tbsp extra-virgin olive oil

Juice of 1 lime

A pinch of chilli flakes

tip

I recommend cooking a little of the batter first as a tester to check seasoning and texture.

These are perfect for a party, picnic or lunchbox. Chickpea flour is brilliant in the batter as it means you can go egg-free. Eggs and cheese are often used in fritters, so it's lovely to have a plant-based version. When you can get fresh corn on the cob, you'll want the kernels from about 2 medium ears of corn, otherwise use defrosted frozen sweetcorn or tinned. Leftover fritters are delicious cold.

Mix all the ingredients for the fritters in a big bowl, except the ghee, seasoning with 1½ teaspoons of salt and ½ teaspoon of black pepper. Scrunch the veg really well as you mix, as this helps to release liquid which gets absorbed by the flour and helps bind the fritters. Stir well and then set aside for about 10 minutes.

Meanwhile, make the herby yoghurt by mixing everything together in a bowl and seasoning to taste with salt and pepper. Next, make the tomato salsa by mixing everything together in another bowl and seasoning with salt and pepper.

Pop the oven on at a low temperature so you can keep the fritters warm as they cook, although they are super delicious cold too.

In large frying pan (big enough to hold four fritters at a time without overcrowding), melt a quarter of the ghee on a medium–high heat so the whole base is covered. Add just under 2 tablespoons of batter for each fritter to the pan – the smaller the fritters, the easier to turn them, and you get crispier edges as a bonus! Fry for 4–5 minutes on the first side and then 3–4 minutes on the second side until golden all over. On the first side use your spatula to apply a bit of pressure on the top, as another way of helping the fritters to stick together before flipping them. Resist trying to flip them sooner as they'll fall apart; turn down the heat if you're worried they might burn, and be gentle as you turn them over.

Repeat with the remaining ghee and batter, popping the finished fritters in the oven to keep warm as you make them, then serve up with the yoghurt and salsa.

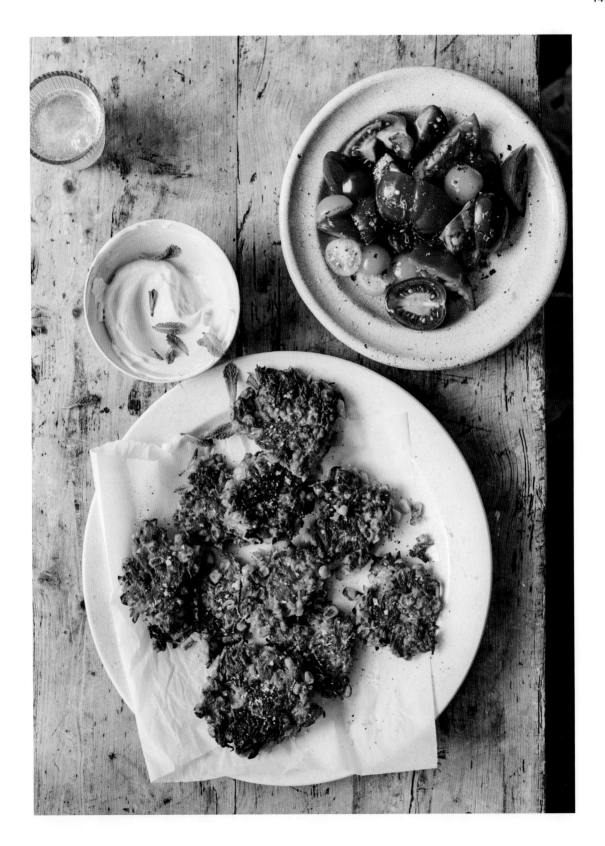

veg powered and plant based

one-pot sweet potato and spinach-lentil bake

feeds 4 ———— 1 hour

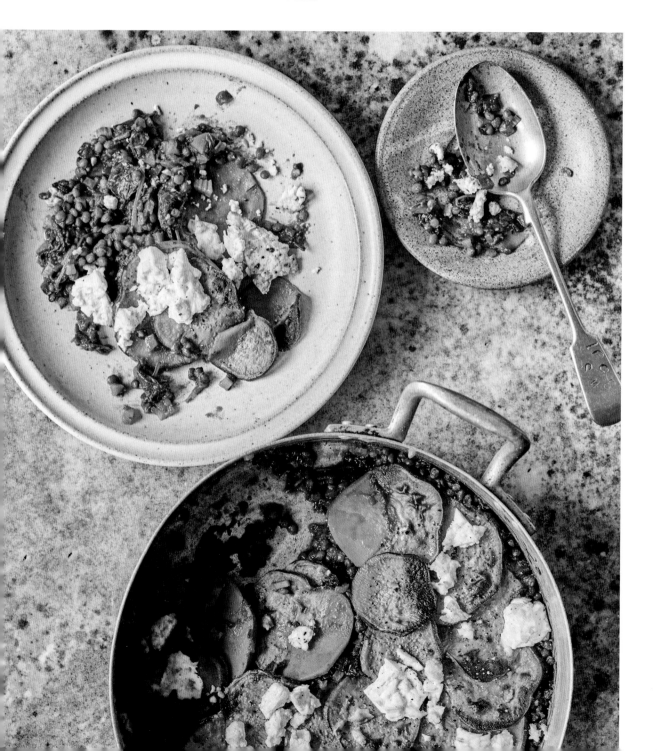

1 tbsp butter, olive oil or ghee

1 large onion, finely diced

1 carrot, scrubbed and finely diced

1 celery stick or 1 small fennel
  bulb, finely diced

3 garlic cloves, finely diced

1 tsp dried thyme or mixed herbs

2 × 400g tins of green or brown
  lentils, drained and rinsed *(480g)*

2 tsp *(rose)* harissa paste
  (or more to taste)

400g tin of chopped tomatoes

300ml veg stock, *plus more
  if needed*

50g feta

300g baby spinach

Sea salt and black pepper

topping

500g sweet potatoes

150g feta

1 handful of fresh parsley or
  coriander, roughly chopped,
  to serve

A hearty one-pot midweek supper, perfect served with lemon-dressed salad leaves. I love bakes with a creamy root-veg mash, but this time I wanted an alternative with more texture (that tasted just as good). Enter sweet potato slices with crumbled feta, which goes golden-edged and lovely. Plus you won't need a second pot to make it – win-win! Look for rose harissa paste – it has a gorgeous sweet smokiness. Brands vary in heat, so if you're cautious, add 1 teaspoon at the start, then taste and adjust before you add the topping.

Preheat the oven to fan 220°C/gas mark 9.

In a wide ovenproof pot with a lid, melt the butter, add the onion and fry on a medium heat for 5 minutes, stirring occasionally, then add the carrot and celery or fennel and cook for another 5 minutes.

Add the garlic, thyme or mixed herbs and a good pinch of sea salt and pepper, and fry for another minute. Stir in the lentils, harissa, tinned tomatoes and stock. Stir everything together well, pop the lid on the pot and bring to the boil, then turn the heat down to a medium simmer and cook for 8 minutes, stirring halfway through.

Scrub the sweet potatoes (no need to peel them) and slice into 3mm-thick rounds, toss them in a little olive oil and sea salt and pepper.

Crumble the 50g feta for the filling into the pot and stir in the spinach and cook for a couple of minutes – keeping the lid on will help it to wilt even faster – then stir and taste for seasoning. If you went easy on the harissa levels, you could always add a little more here. If the lentil and spinach mixture looks a little thick, add a splash more stock; if it looks a bit watery, keep the lid off and simmer away for 3 minutes, letting the liquid reduce.

Next, arrange the sweet potato rounds on top of the lentils, overlapping them a little. Pop into the oven (without the lid) and bake for 10 minutes, then take the pot out and scatter over the feta for the topping, crumbling it as you go. Switch the oven to its grill setting and cook for about another 15 minutes until the sweet potatoes are tender and going golden at the edges and the feta is browning, keeping an eye on them to make sure the edges don't get too dark. Scatter over the fresh herbs to finish.

fried halloumi and chickpea rainbow salad

feeds 2 as a main ——— 15 minutes

2 tbsp ghee or coconut oil

400g tin of chickpeas, drained
  and rinsed

4 tsp garam masala

2 tsp ground cumin

225g halloumi, cut into small cubes

2 tsp maple syrup

Sea salt and pepper

salad

A little diced red onion or
  chopped spring onions

1 large carrot, scrubbed and
  roughly grated

1 handful of diced ripe tomatoes

**cashew-coriander-mint
chutney** *makes double*

4 tbsp cashews or other nuts

4 handfuls of fresh coriander

2 small handful of fresh mint leaves

2 fresh green chilli, descended if
  you prefer, chopped, or a good
  pinch of chilli flakes

½ tsp ground cumin

Juice of 3 limes

4 tbsp olive oil

Definitely make this! It's also delicious stuffed into a wrap, or serve it with rice or quinoa. Halloumi needs to be served straight away, so make this fresh. Swap the halloumi for paneer, or use extra-firm tofu, patted dry, for a plant-based version of this dish.

Prepare the salad and arrange in two bowls.

Heat up a large frying pan and toast the cashews for the chutney on a medium heat for 3–4 minutes, tossing halfway through, until lightly golden, then tip half of them into the small bowl of a food processor and save the rest for garnishing.

Put the pan back on the heat, melt 1½ tablespoons of the ghee and fry the chickpeas (making sure they are dried well in a tea towel before so they don't spit in the hot oil) on a medium heat for 4 minutes with half of the spices and a pinch of salt, stirring every now and then. Tip into a bowl, scraping out the delicious bits from the bottom of the pan as you go.

While the chickpeas are frying, add all the other chutney ingredients to the food processor – saving a few herbs for garnishing, if you like – along with about 3 tablespoons of water, then blend together, seasoning to taste with salt and pepper.

Put the pan back on the heat with the rest of the ghee and, when melted, fry the halloumi on a medium heat for about 2 minutes on the first side on (keep the pieces of halloumi spaced out) and then turn, sprinkle over the rest of the spices and fry for about 1 minute on the other side until lightly golden brown and crispy at the edges. Straight away add the fried chickpeas and the maple syrup, then toss together with the halloumi and fry for 30 seconds so that the chickpeas warm through and the maple syrup bubbles and thickens. Scatter the chickpeas over the bowls of salad with the halloumi on top, drizzle over half of the chutney and top with the remaining nuts.

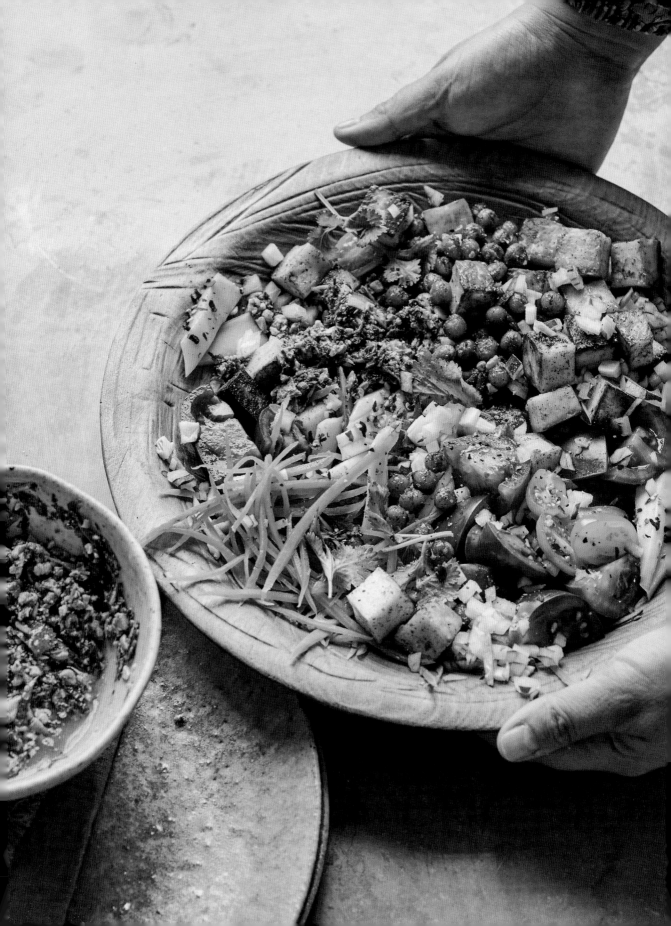

one-pan masala beans with eggs

feeds 2 ——— 25 minutes

1 ½ tbsp coconut oil or ghee
1 medium onion, finely chopped
2 garlic cloves, finely chopped
2 tsp finely grated or finely
  chopped fresh ginger
1 tsp ground coriander
¼ tsp ground turmeric
½ tsp ground cumin
1 fresh chilli, deseeded if you
  prefer and chopped, or a pinch
  of chilli flakes
2 tsp tomato purée
400g tin of chopped tomatoes
  or passata
2 tsp maple syrup or *(coconut)* sugar
400g tin of cannellini or haricot
  beans, drained and rinsed
Sea salt and black pepper

to serve

2 eggs
1 handful of grated Cheddar
1 handful of chopped fresh
  coriander

optional extras

Spicy chutney or natural yoghurt
Squeeze of lime or lemon juice or
  some pickled onion *(page 246)*

An Indian-inspired take on eggs with baked beans – a real favourite! I love it served with homemade chips, either fried or roasted, and see my **Loaded Root Veg Wedges** on page 165 if you'd like to change things up. Also delicious on toast. Swap the spices for 2 teaspoons of curry powder if you like.

Melt the coconut oil in a frying pan, add the onion and cook on a medium heat for 10 minutes until softened, then add the garlic, ginger and spices and a pinch of salt and cook for another 2 minutes, stirring regularly.

Stir in the tomato purée and cook for just under a minute, then add the tinned tomatoes or passata, the maple syrup or sugar and the beans and cook for 10 minutes until thick and reduced. Let it get nice and thick like baked beans and season to taste with salt and pepper.

If you want to keep this in one pan, make two gaps in the beans after they have been cooking for around 5 minutes, crack in the eggs, season with salt and pepper and scatter over the grated cheese. Pop a lid on the pan and cook for 4–5 minutes until the egg whites are set, while the yolks are still runny, and the cheese has melted over the beans. If you prefer, you can fry your eggs instead, just remember to do this when the beans have around 3 minutes left and cook until the egg whites are set.

Serve up straight away scattered with the fresh coriander and topped with any of the optional extras.

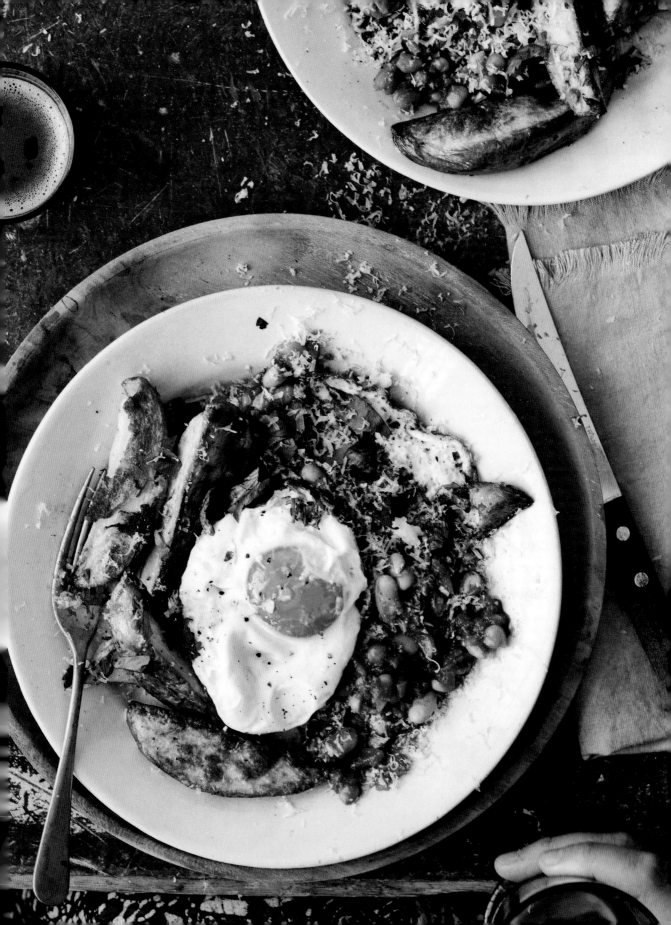

shiitake mushroom adobo

feeds 4 ———— 30 minutes

4–6 tbsp ghee or coconut oil

300g shiitake mushrooms *(or something equally special and firm such as oyster)*, roughly sliced

300g chestnut or button mushrooms, roughly sliced

2 small red onions, diced

4 big garlic cloves, finely chopped

3 bay leaves *(fresh or dried)*

1½–2 tsp black pepper *(to taste)*

5 tbsp tamari or soy sauce

5 tbsp apple cider vinegar

3 tsp coconut sugar

Sea salt

to serve

Coconut Rice *(page 156)*

Some sliced cucumber or 1 big handful of watercress, to serve

optional extras

1 fried egg per person *(if you're feeling hungry!)*

A squeeze of your favourite chilli sauce

The key flavours of Filipino adobo are garlic, vinegar, black pepper, soy sauce and bay leaf. I grew up on chicken adobo. This mushroom version is super delicious and simple. Traditionally, adobo is served with white rice, which I've made extra delicious by cooking in coconut milk – see page 156 – but some of my Filipino aunties (my *Titas*) will tell you that they have adopted quinoa later in life and love it as much as rice (see variation)!

Heat up a large wok or deep-sided frying pan and melt 1 tablespoon of the ghee. Tumble in half of the shiitake mushrooms, add a little pinch of salt, stir to coat in the hot ghee and then fry, undisturbed, on a high heat for 2 minutes before turning and frying for 2 minutes on the other side. Remove from the pan and set aside. Liquid will be released as they fry and the mushrooms will take on a firmer, meatier texture.

Using the same pan, repeat with the rest of the mushrooms, adding a little more ghee, if needed, plus another little pinch of salt, and set aside.

Heat up another tablespoon of the ghee and fry the onion on a medium heat for 4 minutes, then add the garlic and bay leaves and cook for another 3 minutes, stirring regularly.

Add the black pepper, tamari or soy sauce, vinegar and sugar and simmer gently, uncovered, for 5 minutes to thicken and reduce a little, then add the mushrooms and simmer for another 2 minutes. Taste for seasoning: you might want to add a little more pepper.

Remove from the heat and serve with the coconut rice and some sliced cucumber or watercress. I like a fried egg too.

variation

I like to serve this with a mix of rice and quinoa, rinsing both well and cooking together for 15 minutes, lid on, then leaving to sit for 5 minutes (lid still on) before fluffing with a fork.

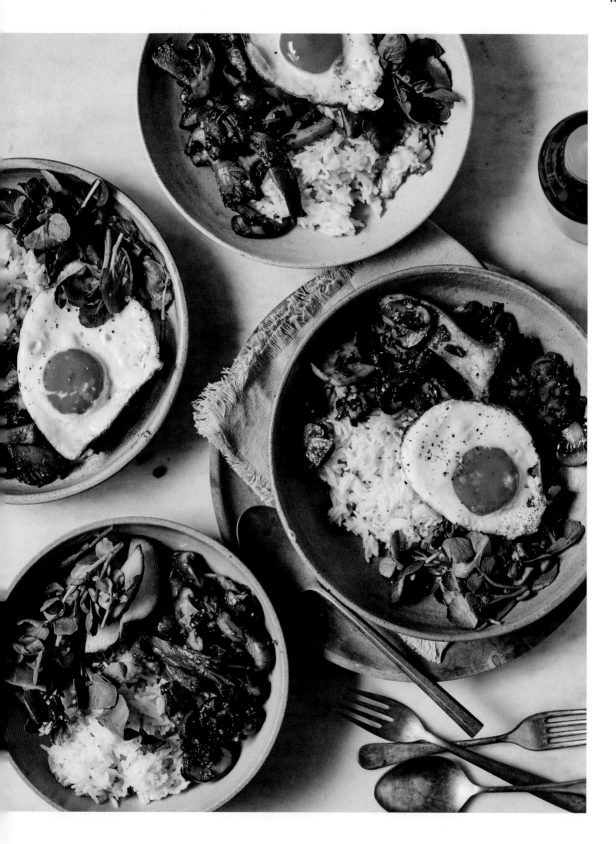

veg powered and plant based

coconut rice

feeds 4 as a side ———— 20 minutes

2 tsp coconut oil or ghee
250g white basmati rice,
   well rinsed
¼ tsp sea salt
400ml tin of coconut milk

optional extras
A few tbsp chopped fresh
   coriander or spring onions
A good squeeze of lime or
   lemon juice
2 tsp tamari or soy sauce
A pinch of chilli flakes

Delicious served with the **Shiitake Mushroom Adobo** on page 154. I've used white basmati rice here, but you could swap for brown basmati or quinoa (see variation). If the cooked rice appears too wet for your liking, simply take the lid off the pan and leave it to dry out for a minute or two on the hob on the lowest heat setting.

Melt the coconut oil in a medium saucepan on a medium heat. Add the rice and salt and stir well to coat it in the hot oil. Cook for a minute.

Turn up the heat. Add the coconut milk, then stir well, pop a lid on the pan and bring to the boil. Immediately reduce the heat to a low simmer without removing the lid (as steam will escape and cooking will be disrupted).

After 8 minutes of simmering, check if the rice needs more water. If it does, add a few tablespoons of hot water. Cook for another 4 minutes (12 minutes in total) until all the liquid has been absorbed, then remove from the heat, with the lid still on the pan, and let it sit for 5 minutes.

Serve as a side with your choice of extras sprinkled on top.

pictured on page 155

variation

If using brown basmati rice or quinoa, add 50–100ml hot water with the coconut milk and cook for an extra 8–10 minutes or until tender. If using quinoa, fluff with a fork before serving.

veg kebabs Filipino-style

makes 8 medium skewers ———— 35 minutes

2 handfuls of mushrooms
(see introduction)

1 red onion or 6 spring onions,
sliced into small chunks

2 peppers *(orange and red)*,
deseeded and sliced
into 2.5cm chunks

2 small courgettes, sliced into
1cm chunks

8 baby sweetcorn, sliced in half
lengthways to make 16 pieces

8 cherry tomatoes

200g paneer or halloumi *(patted
dry)*, sliced into 16 cubes

2 tbsp melted ghee or coconut
oil, for brushing

Mango-Tomato Salsa *(page 179)*,
to serve

Filipino-style sauce

4 tbsp apple cider vinegar

2 tbsp tamari or soy sauce

2 tsp–1 tbsp fish sauce *(to taste
– vegan if you prefer)* or extra
tamari or soy sauce

2 tbsp *(coconut)* sugar or maple
syrup

2 star anise or ½ tsp Chinese
five-spice powder

¼ tsp chilli flakes *(or to taste)*

3 garlic cloves, finely chopped

Sea salt and black pepper

My Filipino mum inspired this recipe as the sauce is fantastic in stir-fries and also makes veg kebabs anything but boring. I've really enjoyed expanding my mushroom horizons and changing them up as each type is unique, so for this I'd go for 2 large portobello mushrooms, sliced into eighths, or 12 oyster or button mushrooms. If you can get two types of mushroom on your skewer, all the better, and if you have any cooked small new potatoes, add these too. Serve with the **Mango-Tomato Salsa** on page 179.

———————————————————————

If you don't have reusable skewers, soak bamboo or wooden skewers in water for at least 30 minutes before you make your kebabs, to prevent them from burning during cooking. If using a barbecue, get it going now!

Mix all the sauce ingredients together in a large mixing bowl and add a little pinch of sea salt (as the tamari/soy and fish sauce are already quite salty) and some pepper. Do this step ahead, if you have time.

Add all the veg and the paneer or halloumi to the bowl and toss them in the sauce. Leave to marinate for 20 minutes while the skewers are soaking and while the barbecue (if using) is heating up.

Thread the veg and paneer or halloumi onto the soaked skewers, alternating the mushrooms and other veg with the cubes of cheese.

Brush the barbecue grate or a griddle pan (set on a medium heat) with the melted ghee, then cook the skewers for 5 minutes on one side before turning over and cooking on the other side for another 4–5 minutes until the veg are just tender and the edges are going golden and getting charred in places. Remove from the heat and serve up on a big platter with **Mango-Tomato Salsa** (page 179).

pictured on page 180

mushroom and aubergine pancakes with sesame sauce

feeds 4 ———— 35 minutes

pancake filling

2 tbsp coconut oil

400g mixed mushrooms *(250g chestnut and 150g shiitake/oyster)*

2 small-to-medium aubergines

1½ tsp Chinese five-spice powder

2 tsp toasted sesame oil

Sea salt and black pepper

sesame sauce

3 tbsp tahini or smooth nut butter *(stirred well in the jar first)*

5 tbsp tamari or soy sauce

1½ tbsp maple syrup

3 tbsp orange juice

1½ tsp toasted sesame oil

1 tsp Chinese five-spice powder

2 garlic cloves, finely chopped

to serve

1 cucumber, sliced into matchsticks

6 spring onions, sliced into matchsticks

12 small shop-bought Chinese-style pancakes or wraps

Leaves from 2 Little Gem lettuces

This hoisin-inspired sauce, made thick and creamy with tahini, is a favourite of mine. I've been making it for over 10 years since I was private cheffing for bands, who loved duck pancakes. This is a plant-based homage to that classic. King oyster, oyster and shiitake mushrooms work well here, if you can get them, and portobello or chestnut are fantastic too. The ingredients list looks a little long, but a few of the same ingredients are used in the filling and the sauce.

Preheat oven to fan 190°C/gas mark 6½, then divide the coconut oil between two large roasting trays and place in the oven to heat up.

Meanwhile, wipe the mushrooms with a damp tea towel (rather than washing), then roughly slice, keeping small ones whole. If you're using king oyster mushrooms, shred the stems with a fork. Slice the aubergines into thin wedges so that they can cook in the same amount of time as the mushrooms.

Once the coconut oil has melted, transfer the mushrooms to one tray and aubergines to the other, divide the Chinese five-spice and toasted sesame oil between them, along with a good pinch of salt and pepper, and toss well. Spread the veg in an even layer in each tray and roast for 25 minutes, tossing halfway through and swapping the trays so that whichever was on top goes in the middle, and vice versa.

Meanwhile, mix together all the ingredients for the sauce in a small bowl. Add a teaspoon or so of warm water to make the sauce looser, if you like, and season to taste.

Place the cucumber, spring onions, herbs, lettuce and pancakes on a serving dish in separate piles. Warm up the pancakes according to the packet instructions, then serve up with the filling, sauce and salad items, letting everyone assemble their pancakes as they like. Use the lettuce leaves instead of pancakes, if you like.

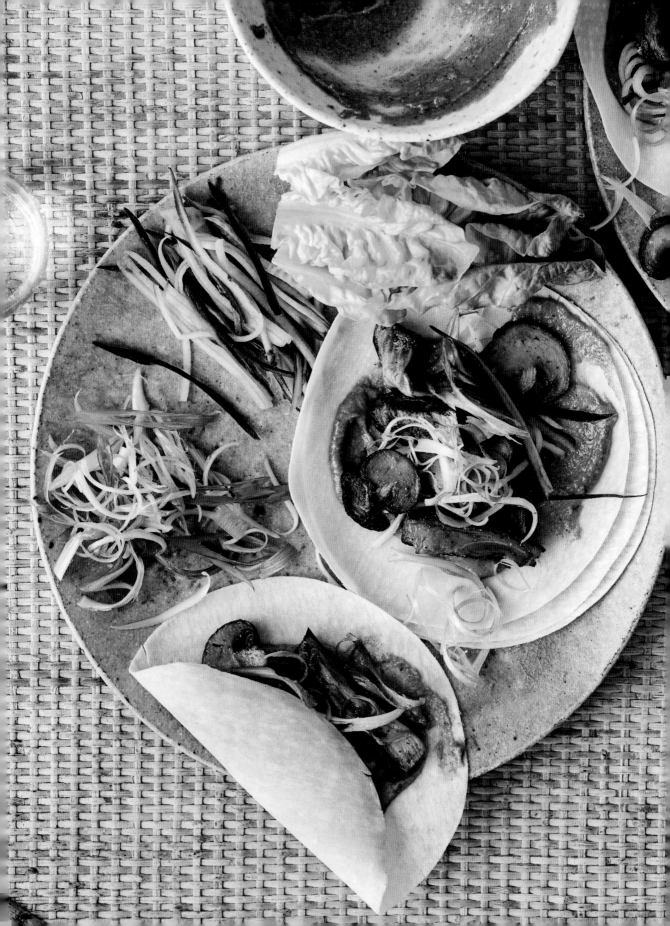

roast carrots and fresh beetroot with dukkah and herby bean dip

feeds 4 as a side ———— 40 minutes

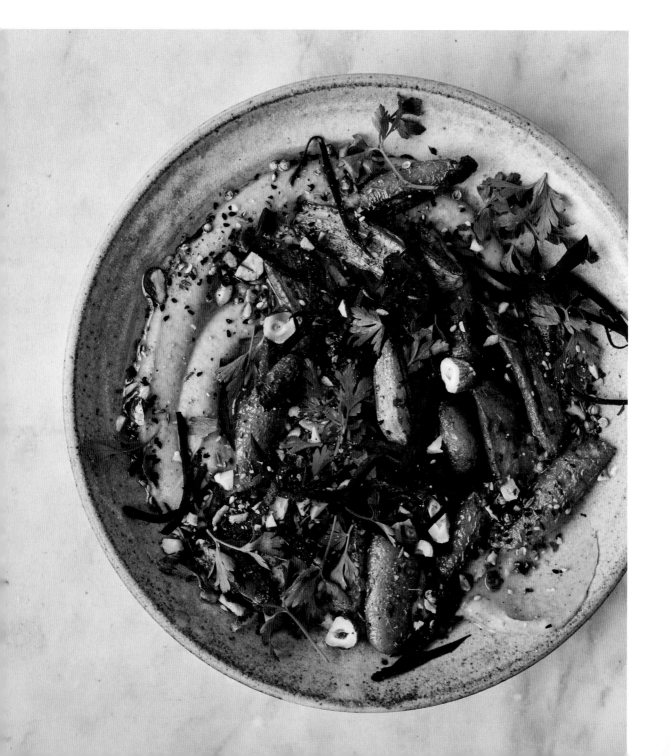

2 tbsp ghee or coconut oil

6 large carrots *(about 400g)*

1 tsp dried or 2 sprigs of
fresh thyme or rosemary

2 small beetroot *(purple or
multicoloured)*

Sea salt and black pepper

dukkah *makes triple*

60g mixed nuts *(such as hazelnuts,
almonds, cashews and walnuts)*

1 tsp cumin seeds

1½ tsp coriander seeds

½ tsp fennel seeds

4 tbsp mixed sesame seeds

herby bean dip

400g tin of white beans or
chickpeas, drained and rinsed

1 large handful of fresh herbs
(such as parsley or coriander), plus
extra to garnish

1 jalapeño or other fresh chilli,
deseeded if you prefer, halved

1 large garlic clove

Juice and grated zest of 1 lemon

2 tbsp extra-virgin olive oil, plus
extra for drizzling

This is on regular rotation at my place during the winter. I make this with a few handfuls of quinoa or lentils and enjoy it hot or warm. I love the contrast between the roasted carrots and the fresh and crunchy raw beetroot. The dukkah recipe makes extra – perfect to keep for sprinkling on salads and soups. Hazelnuts are included in the traditional Egyptian recipe, but I often use a mix of nuts.

Preheat the oven to fan 220°C/gas mark 9, then place the ghee in a large roasting tray and pop in the oven to heat up.

Meanwhile, scrub the carrots (I don't bother peeling them) and dry well in a clean tea towel. Roughly chop at a slight angle, then toss with a good pinch of salt and pepper in the hot ghee and spread out in the roasting tray in a single layer. Place in the oven and roast for 20 minutes.

Pull the tray out, toss the carrots with the herbs and roast for another 10–15 minutes until tender and going golden at the edges.

Meanwhile, make the dukkah. Toast the nuts for about 3 minutes in a large frying pan on a medium heat, then shake the pan, add the spices and toast for another 2 minutes until the nuts are lightly golden and the spices are fragrant. Roughly chop and mix in a bowl, or use a pestle and mortar. Put the pan back on the heat and toast the sesame seeds for another 2–3 minutes, then tip them into the rest of the dukkah mix and add a big pinch of salt and pepper.

Next, make the dip. Place all the ingredients for the dip into a food processor together with 1–3 tablespoons of cold water, then blitz until smooth and season with salt and pepper to taste.

Peel the beetroot and finely slice into matchsticks, washing your hands and board straight away to avoid staining.

Spread and smear the dip onto a large serving plate. Once the carrots are ready, scatter them over the dip, followed by the beetroot matchsticks, drizzle with a little olive oil and then scatter over roughly a third of the dukkah (about 3 tablespoons) and the extra herbs.

shawarma-inspired cauliflower and sweet potato bowls

feeds 2 —————— 35 minutes

2 tbsp ghee, coconut or olive oil
½ cauliflower *(about 400g)*
1 large sweet potato, scrubbed
2 garlic cloves, finely chopped
Grated zest of ½ lemon
Sea salt and black pepper
Tahini Yoghurt *(page 166 – minus the lime / lemon juice)*, to serve

spice mix
½ tsp ground cinnamon
1 tsp ground coriander
1 tsp ground cumin
1 tsp ground turmeric
A pinch of chilli flakes or ⅛ tsp cayenne pepper *(or to taste)*
1 tsp smoked paprika

salad
Shredded cabbage or lettuce
Grated carrot
Chopped tomatoes

optional extras
Sliced red onion or pickled onions *(page 246)*
1 lemon, sliced into wedges
Quick-pickled Veg *(page 246)* or chilli sauce *(optional)*

This is a simple recipe that takes only half an hour to make, or less if you use a shop-bought shawarma spice mix, but I hope you'll give the homemade one a whirl when you have time. Enjoy this with chickpeas, rice or quinoa and some of the veg topping options, or serve with wraps or naan bread. It's also delicious with the **Mango-Tomato Salsa** (page 179), **Coriander-Lime Drizzle** (page 203) or **Spicy Mayo** (page 246). This makes a great packed lunch.

Preheat the oven to fan 220°C/gas mark 9, then place the ghee in a large roasting tray and pop in the oven to melt.

Meanwhile, mix the spices together in a big bowl. Cut the cauliflower into even-sized florets and the sweet potato into wedges and mix in the bowl with the melted ghee, spices, garlic, lemon zest and some salt and pepper. Stir to coat well and set aside.

Once the oven is hot, tip the spice-coated cauliflower and sweet potato onto the hot tray, spread out in a single layer and roast in oven for 25–30 minutes until the veg are tender and going golden at the edges, tossing when it is two-thirds of the way through the roasting time.

Divide the salad between two bowls, add the cauliflower and sweet potato and serve with the tahini yoghurt and topped with any of the optional extras.

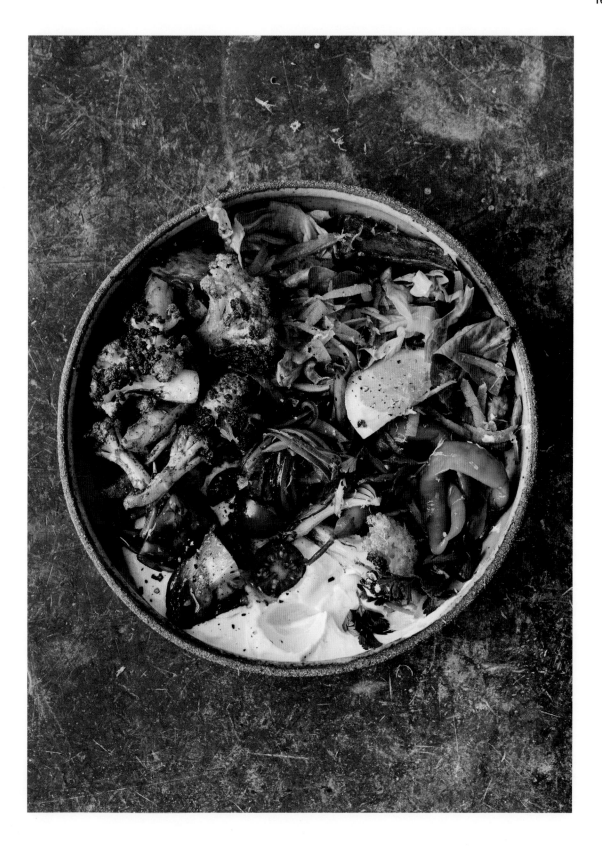

veg powered and plant based

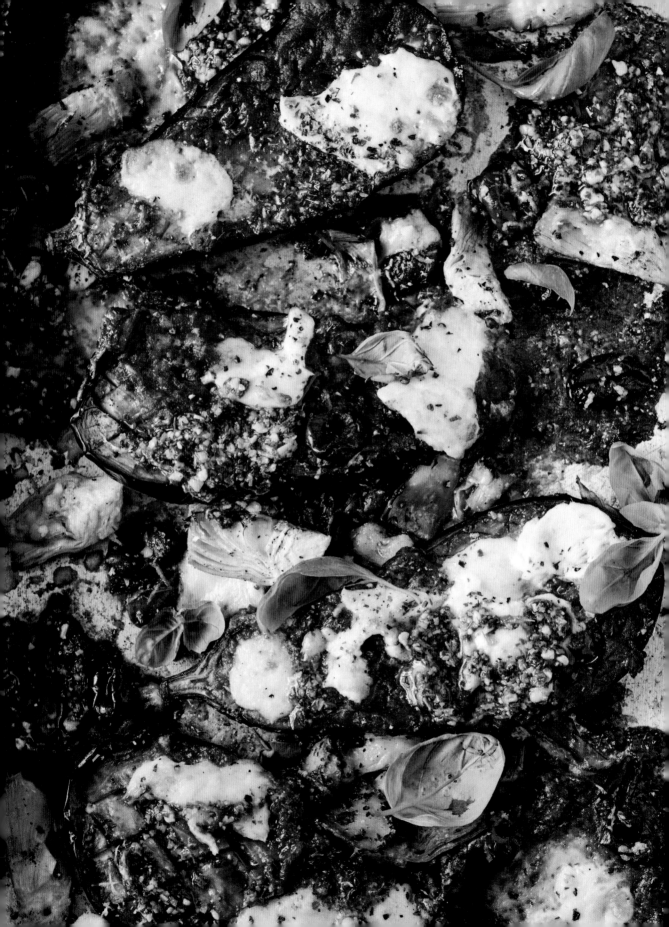

pesto-mozzarella
baked aubergines

feeds 2 ———— 40 minutes

2 medium aubergines

2 tbsp extra-virgin olive oil or
melted butter

150ml thick tomato pasta sauce
*(shop-bought or make your own
– see page 120)*

1 tsp dried oregano or Italian-
style mixed herbs

A pinch of chilli flakes *(optional)*

200g mozzarella, drained well
and sliced

2 tbsp pesto *(shop-bought or make
your own – see page 123)*

1 handful of *(black)* olives, pitted
and torn in half

Sea salt and black pepper

Fresh basil leaves, to serve

optional extras

Chopped sun-dried tomatoes

Anchovies or capers

A drizzle of chilli oil

1 handful of toasted pine nuts

1 handful of toasted
breadcrumbs

Here we have everyone's favourite pizza ingredients baked onto aubergines! Everything happens on one big tray in the oven so it's super simple to put together. Let everyone help themselves, topping their aubergine boats exactly as they like them. Serve with a big salad and some garlic bread or **Farinata** (page 218).

Preheat the oven to fan 220°C/gas mark 9.

Slice the aubergines in half lengthways, then score the flesh on the diagonal in each direction – this will help them to soak up the sauce and to cook and soften more quickly. Rub the scored aubergine flesh with the olive oil and some salt and pepper, then place on a baking tray, flesh side up, and roast for 18 minutes.

Divide the tomato sauce between the aubergine halves and sprinkle with the oregano or mixed herbs and the chilli flakes, if you like. Add the mozzarella, sprinkle it with a little salt and then dollop over the pesto and scatter with the olives and any extras.

Bake in the oven for 15 minutes and finish off under a hot grill for a final 3–5 minutes for the mozzarella to get golden on top. Once out of the oven, scatter over the basil leaves.

loaded root veg wedges with *mojo verde* and tahini yoghurt

feeds 4 as a side ——— 40 minutes

2 tbsp ghee or coconut oil
800g mix of carrots, parsnips
  and potatoes
Sea salt and black pepper
2 tbsp mixed sesame seeds,
  to serve

mojo verde *makes extra*
1 tsp ground cumin or
  ½ tsp cumin seeds
2 garlic cloves, peeled
2 handfuls of fresh coriander
2 handfuls of fresh parsley
1 fresh green chilli, deseeded
  and roughly chopped
2 tbsp lime or lemon juice
4 tbsp extra-virgin olive oil

tahini yoghurt
100g Greek-style yoghurt
2 tbsp tahini *(stirred well in
  the jar first)*
1 garlic clove, finely chopped
2 tbsp lime or lemon juice

I can't get enough of Spanish *mojo verde*. It's one of my favourite green sauces – perfect with salads and soups or to perk up roasted or grilled veg. Here I've used carrots, potatoes and parsnips, which go crispier than sweet potatoes, but sweet potatoes, while less crispy, are still delicious. The toppings look fantastic dolloped and drizzled over but to keep the wedges crispy for longer, you could serve the tahini yoghurt on the side with a swirl of *mojo verde* on top.

———

Preheat the oven to fan 220°C/gas mark 9, then place the ghee in one very large roasting tray or two medium ones and pop in the oven to heat up.

Scrub the veg well (without peeling) and slice into wedges 7–8cm in length and either 2.5cm wide for the carrots and parsnips or 1cm wide for the potatoes. This way they'll all roast in around the same length of same time. Toss them carefully in the hot ghee, season with salt and pepper and spread out in a single layer in the tray(s), then roast for 20 minutes. Remove from the oven, toss in the tray(s) (swapping them round, if using two trays, so that the veg all cook evenly) and roast for another 10 minutes.

Meanwhile, toast the cumin for a minute or two in a hot pan, then add to a food processor with all the other ingredients for the *mojo verde*. Add 2 tablespoons of water and blitz until chunkily combined, then season to taste with salt and pepper.

Mix the tahini yoghurt ingredients together in a bowl and season to taste with salt and pepper.

As soon as the veg are out the oven, dollop over the *mojo verde* and tahini yoghurt, scatter with the sesame seeds and serve straight away while hot. The toppings cool the veg down fast, so it's very much a 'Let's dig in now!'.

feel good

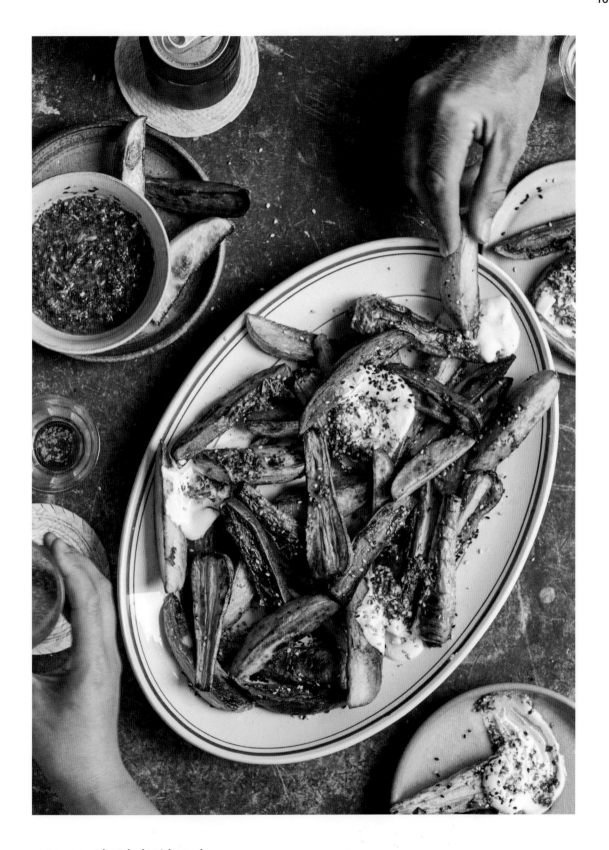

veg powered and plant based

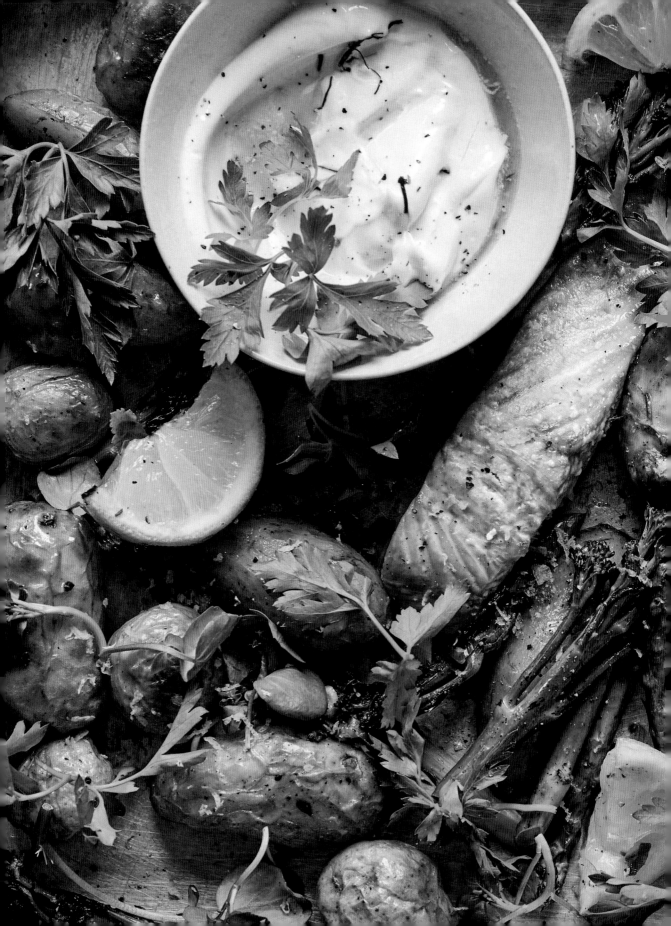

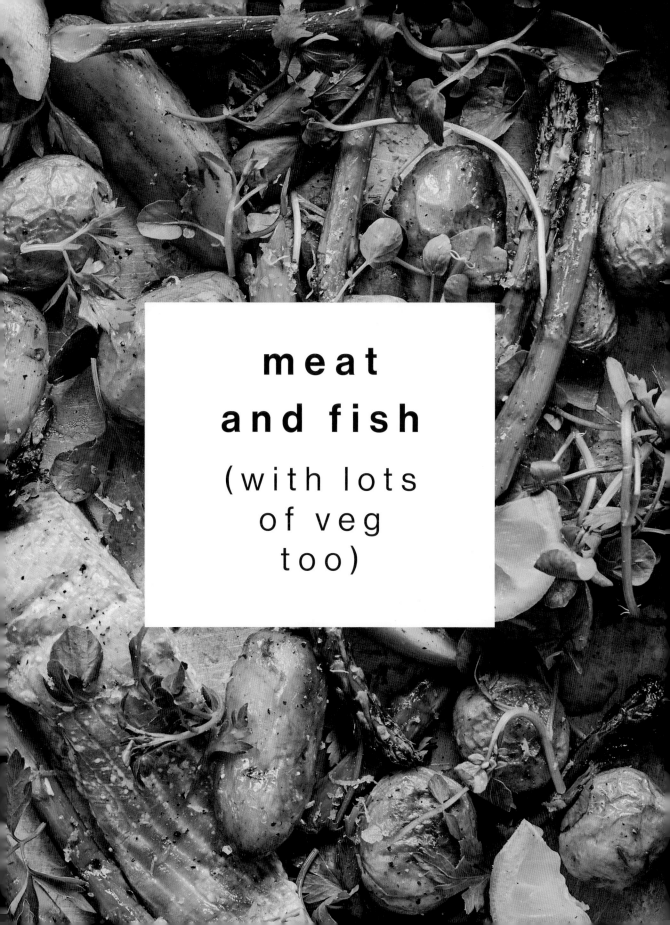

meat and fish

(with lots of veg too)

/ when it comes to meat and fish, buy the best you can source /

When it comes to meat and fish, I recommend buying the best you can source and allow for in your shopping budget. Better quality does make it more expensive, but I try to balance this by buying less and eating it less frequently. If you haven't got a good butcher or fishmonger near you, have a look online as you can order direct from top-quality producers around the country and then store the fish or meat in the freezer to use as needed, which is a good way of avoiding waste as well as supporting small suppliers.

In the recipes in this chapter, you'll find that at least two-thirds of each dish will still be made up of vegetables and other ingredients so that your meat or fish goes further. A great example is the **Fishcakes** (page 195), where sweet potatoes, peas and herbs help a relatively conservative amount of fish go a long way while still providing a delicious and hearty meal.

Many of the recipes in this chapter can also be tweaked to make them suitable for plant-based eaters. For a vegetarian version of the **Spiced Feta-Meatball Traybake** (page 174), for instance, use the **Veg Balls** (page 120) instead. Similarly, the **Half-and-Half Cottage Pie with Cheesy Parsnip Mash** (page 176) could be made fully veggie with 100 per cent lentils.

If you love fish, don't miss the following recipes from other chapters, such as the **Fish Finger Tacos with Avocado Cream** (page 211) or, with oily fish in particular being recommended by health experts, why not try the **Smoked Mackerel Pâté** (page 82) or the **Store-cupboard Sardine Puttanesca with Tagliatelle** (page 126) – two of my favourites. If you have 15 minutes to whip up a dinner for friends, then do give the **Crab and Courgette Spaghetti** (page 112) a go. Fresh-tasting from the chilli, lemon and herbs, it feels special even though the dish comes together in a flash.

spicy fish with coriander and lime quinoa and simple salsa

feeds 2 ———— 25 minutes

120g quinoa, rinsed
400g tin of black beans,
  drained and rinsed
1 tbsp ghee or coconut oil
2 fish fillets *(ask your
  fishmonger what's in season)*
¾ tsp smoked paprika
A pinch of chilli flakes
2 tsp lime juice
Lime wedges, to serve

simple salsa
2 ripe tomatoes, diced
1 big handful of finely chopped
  red cabbage
1 tbsp extra-virgin olive oil
Sea salt and black pepper

green sauce
4 spring onions
20g fresh coriander, stems included
1 garlic clove, peeled
8 tbsp extra-virgin olive oil
Juice of 1 lime *(save a little
  squeeze for the salsa)*
A pinch of chilli flakes

Inspired by a trip to Mexico, this lovely fresh green sauce instantly perks me up and makes my kitchen feel sunnier on grey days. The whole recipe is quick enough to put together for a midweek meal and friends love it. For veggie friends, I like to rub the spices into sweet potato wedges or corn on the cob and grill them in place of the fish. The quinoa can be swapped for rice or buckwheat, if you prefer.

Start by making the salsa. Mix the tomatoes and the cabbage in a bowl with the olive oil, salt, pepper and a squeeze of lime (steal it from the green sauce ingredients) and set aside.

Blitz all the green sauce ingredients together in a food processor, seasoning with salt and pepper to taste.

Place the quinoa in a saucepan with 250ml of water and a pinch of salt and cook, covered with a lid, for around 18 minutes (or according to the packet instructions). After 17 minutes, remove the lid, scatter the black beans on top and cook, covered, for a final minute. Remove the pan from the heat and leave to stand.

Heat the ghee in a frying pan on a high heat, then place the fish fillets in the pan, spaced apart and skin side down. Scatter over the spices and a pinch of salt and pepper, using the back of a spoon to pat them into the fish, then tip your pan so you can spoon over a little of the hot ghee or oil. Once the fish has had 3 minutes on one side and it comes away easily, carefully turn, lower the heat a little and cook for another few minutes until the flesh is just cooked through.

Meanwhile, gently stir the beans into the quinoa, along with half the green sauce, taste, then divide between two plates and add a generous spoonful of salsa to each. Top with the fish as soon it's ready and serve with the remaining green sauce alongside.

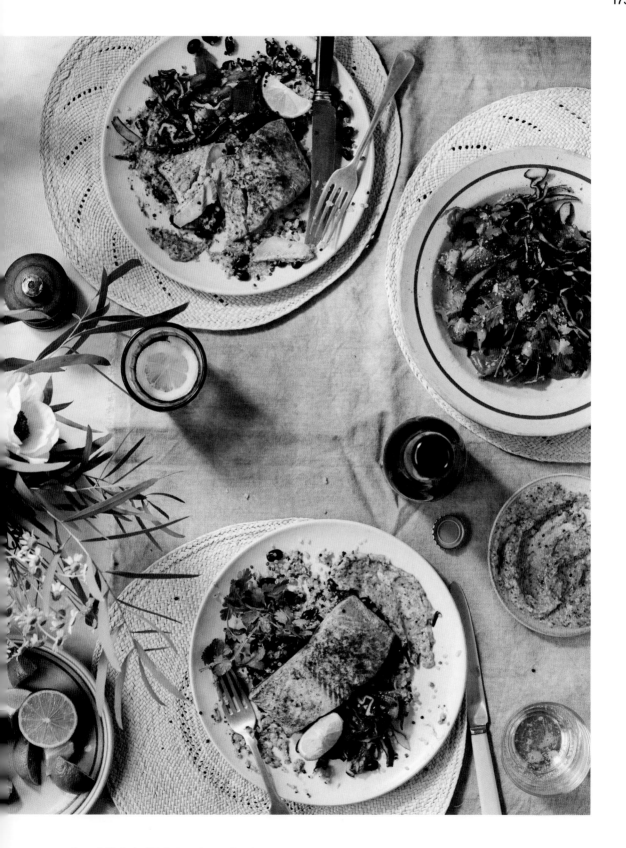

meat and fish (with lots of veg too)

spiced feta-meatball traybake

feeds 4 ———— 45 minutes

400g tin of chickpeas, drained
  and rinsed and dried well
3 potatoes or sweet potatoes,
  scrubbed and cut into wedges
2 peppers, deseeded and
  roughly chopped
2 tbsp oil of your choice or
  melted ghee

spice mix
1½ tsp ground cumin
1 tsp ground turmeric
1 tsp ground coriander
1 heaped tsp dried oregano,
  thyme or rosemary
A pinch of chilli flakes
¾ tsp sea salt
½ tsp black pepper

meatballs
500g minced meat of your choice
100g feta, crumbled
2 garlic cloves, finely chopped
1 egg, beaten
1 red onion, finely diced

yoghurt sauce
100g natural yoghurt
1 small garlic clove, finely
  chopped

to serve
1 handful of fresh mint, parsley
  or dill *(or a mixture)*
½ cucumber, diced
2 medium ripe tomatoes, diced
1 lemon, cut into 4 wedges

Who doesn't love a traybake?! Make sure you scoop out all the delicious spiced juices from the baking tray. The yoghurt sauce is refreshing, so don't skip it. If you're in a hurry, swap the spice mix for a tablespoon of harissa paste or a ras el hanout spice mix. For a veggie version, use the **Veg Balls** on page 120.

Preheat the oven to fan 220°C/gas mark 9 and place a very large roasting tray (or 2 medium ones) into the oven to heat up.

Meanwhile, mix together all the ingredients for the spice mix in a small bowl. In a medium bowl, mix the chickpeas, vegetables and oil with half the spice mix and toss to coat.

Tip the spice-coated chickpeas and vegetables into the heated roasting tray(s) and spread out in a single layer. You want everything to be well spaced apart so that they roast rather than steam. Pop into the oven to roast for 25 minutes.

Meanwhile, add all the ingredients for the meatballs to the medium bowl (no need to clean it out), reserving half of the diced onion for later. Add the remaining spice mix and use a fork to mix everything together. Divide the meatball mixture into 20 balls, rolling each one between your hands, and placing on a large plate.

Remove the chickpeas and vegetables from the oven (after cooking for 25 minutes) and toss together. Spread out on the roasting tray(s) again and nestle the meatballs in the spaces between the veg. Pop back into the oven to roast for another 18–20 minutes, depending on the type of mince you have used. To check, remove one meatball and open it up to make sure that it's cooked through.

While the meatballs are cooking, chop the herbs and combine them in a bowl with chopped cucumber and tomatoes, reserved onion and a pinch of salt and pepper. Mix the yoghurt sauce, seasoning to taste with salt and pepper and finishing with a generous drizzle of olive oil. Squeeze a lemon wedge over the meatballs, roasted veg and salad, and serve with the yoghurt sauce and extra lemon wedges.

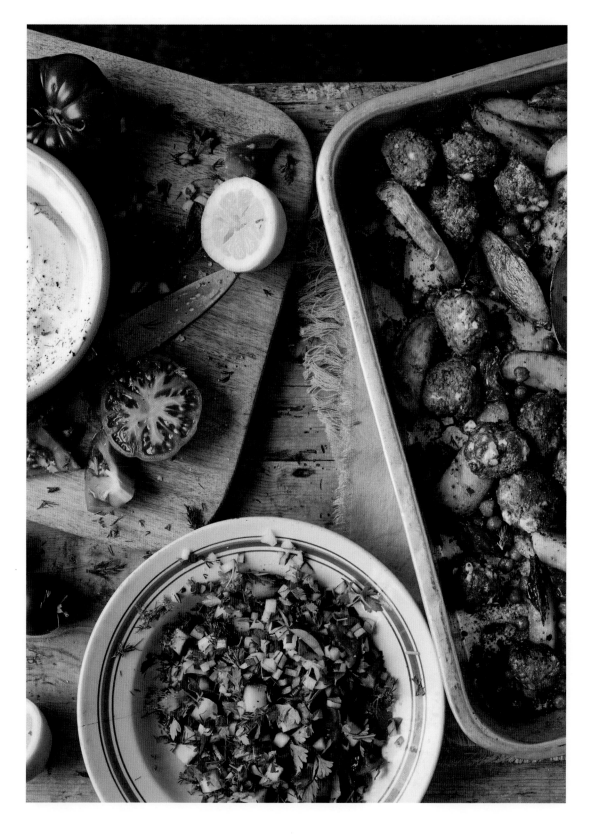

meat and fish (with lots of veg too)

half-and-half cottage pie with cheesy parsnip mash

feeds 4 ———— 1 hour *(hands-on time 40 minutes)*

3 tbsp ghee, butter or olive oil

2 large onions or 1 onion plus
  1 leek, finely chopped

2 celery sticks, diced

3 large carrots, diced

3 garlic cloves, finely chopped

1 tbsp mixed dried herbs or
  2 tbsp chopped fresh herbs
  (such as thyme or rosemary)

250g minced meat *(or a plant-based
  alternative)*

1 tbsp flour *(plain, buckwheat or
  chickpea/gram)*

2 tbsp tomato purée or 1 tbsp
  tomato ketchup

1 tbsp tamari or soy sauce or
  2 tsp Worcestershire sauce

400ml veg or chicken stock,
  plus more if needed

400g tin of green or brown lentils,
  drained and rinsed

Sea salt and black pepper

parsnip mash

1.3kg mix of parsnips and
  potatoes *(about 6 large in total)*,
  chopped into chunks

100ml milk

2 handfuls of grated mature
  Cheddar

1 tbsp chopped herbs *(such as
  parsley or chives)*, for sprinkling
  (optional)

This pan of comfort gets made twice a month without fail as soon as the cold weather kicks in. The filling is half minced meat and half lentils, but of course you can use a plant-based mince or all lentils if you like; swap the meat for another tin of lentils. The pie is veg packed and I love the parsnip mash on top – more parsnip than potato, ratio wise, being my preference. If you've bought organic potatoes, parsnips and carrots, no need to peel them. This reheats well – enjoy it on the weekend and then reheat in the oven for a zero-effort dinner in the week. Serve with a big bowl of buttered peas or broccoli.

Heat up 2 tablespoons of the ghee in a large ovenproof saucepan, add the onions (or onion and leek) and fry on a medium heat for 8 minutes, stirring from time to time.

Add the celery, carrots, garlic and herbs and a big pinch of salt and pepper, then fry for 5 minutes, stirring occasionally and scraping the bottom of the pan. You want the veg to soften and go golden at the edges but not get overly browned.

Push the veg to one side of the pan, then add the remaining tablespoon of ghee. Add the minced meat to the empty part of the pan, turn up the heat a little and fry for 5 minutes, letting the meat break up and brown in parts. You don't need to worry too much about the browning process, but if you've got time, be a bit more leisurely here! Sprinkle salt and pepper over the mince as it browns.

Next, add the flour and stir into the mince and veg. Cook for a few minutes before adding the tomato purée and the tamari or Worcestershire sauce (which will add an amazing depth of flavour) and stirring it all together.

continued overleaf

feel good

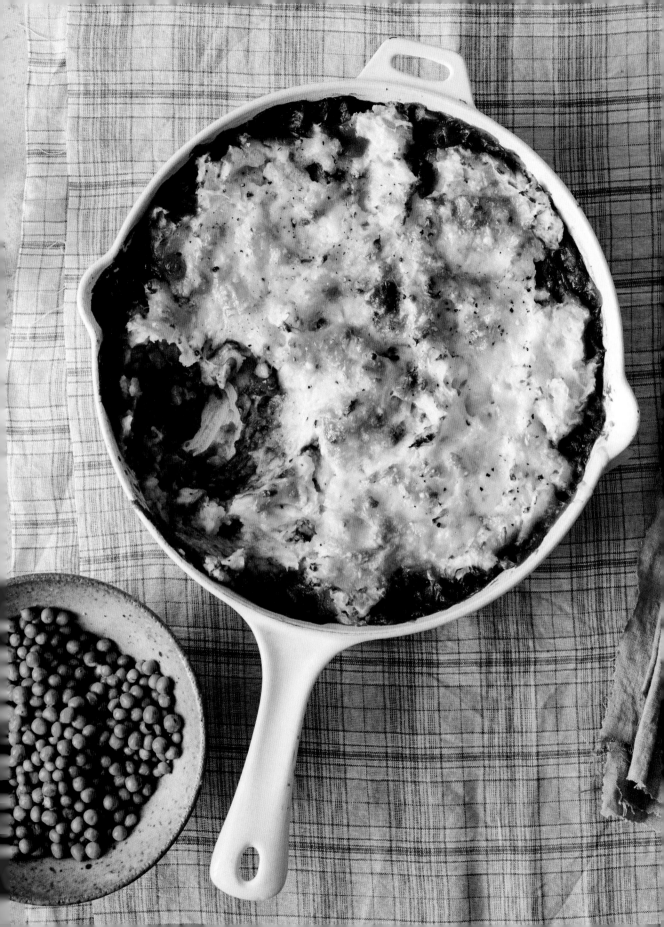

Turn the heat right up, pour in the stock, stirring well and scraping the bottom of the pan to incorporate any flavoursome sticky bits, then add the lentils and simmer for about 25 minutes until the veg are tender and you have a beautiful thick sauce. Season with salt and pepper to taste. If the sauce is reducing too quickly and drying out, add a little more stock and pop a lid on the pan.

Meanwhile, preheat the oven to fan 220°C/gas mark 9 and prepare the mash for the topping. Tip the parsnip and potato chunks into a pan of boiling salted water and strongly simmer for about 20 minutes until tender, then drain and pop back in the pot to steam dry for a few minutes. Roughly mash with a potato masher or fork – I prefer a chunky texture – then stir in the milk and season to taste with salt and pepper.

Top the meat and lentil mixture with the mash. I like it nice and rustic, so I use two spoons to add big dollops of mash, starting from the centre and working outwards. Sprinkle over the grated cheese and bake for 20 minutes. If the top of the pie isn't golden, heat the grill to high and grill for a final 5 minutes, or turn the oven up to 240°C for a final 10 minutes. Finish with a sprinkling of herbs, if you like.

If you can bear to wait, allow the dish to sit for 10 minutes before serving up.

variations

For a plant-based version, try nutritional yeast instead of grated cheese, use dairy-free milk and a vegan Worcestershire sauce.

For a Mexican-style flavour, add 1 teaspoon dried oregano, 1 tablespoon ground cumin and a pinch of chilli flakes, swap the lentils for a tin of kidney beans or mixed beans, and swap the potatoes for sweet potatoes.

Mum's Filipino chicken with mango-tomato salsa

feeds 4 ———— 30 minutes

4 large chicken thighs, skin on
   and bone in *(about 600g)*
Sea salt and black pepper
2 spring onions, finely sliced
   at an angle, to serve

Filipino-style sauce
3 garlic cloves, finely chopped
4 tbsp apple cider vinegar
2 tbsp tamari or soy sauce
2 tsp–1 tbsp fish sauce or 2 tsp
   extra tamari or soy sauce
2 tbsp *(coconut)* sugar or maple
   syrup
2 star anise
¼ tsp chilli flakes *(or to taste)*

mango-tomato salsa
1 big handful of fresh coriander
100g cherry tomatoes, quarterd
100g peeled ripe mango,
   pineapple or stone fruit, diced
2cm fresh ginger, finely grated
½ garlic clove, finely grated
1 jalapeño or other chilli,
   deseeded and diced
Juice of 1 ½ limes
4 spring onions or 1 small red
   onion, finely diced
2 tbsp extra-virgin olive oil
A dash of hot sauce *(optional)*

My mum calls this 'any way chicken' because you can make the chicken any way: I like cooking it in the oven (so I can forget about it); my mum likes to make it on the hob (to keep more of the sauce); and my boyfriend Henry likes grilling it on the barbecue (so it's smoky and crispy). However you do it, I recommend making extra so that you can shred it into soups, wraps, noodles and salads later in the week. This sauce is fantastic in its own right and you'll see it used with vegetables on page 157 too. If you have time to marinate the chicken in the sauce overnight, go for it, but I often forget and just cook it straight away.

Preheat the oven to fan 220°C/gas mark 9. If using a barbecue, get it going now.

Mix all the sauce ingredients together. Place the chicken thighs in an ovenproof dish big enough to arrange the pieces about 2cm apart (but not so big that you lose all the sauce as it cooks off in the oven), then add the sauce, coating each piece of chicken well in the mixture and leave for a few minutes, if you like.

Place the chicken thighs skin-side up in the dish, sprinkle a little salt and pepper over each one and roast for 25 minutes or until well cooked and the juices run clear when pierced with a knife.

Meanwhile, make the salsa. Roughly chop the leaves of the coriander and finely chop the stalks, then add to a serving bowl with all the other ingredients, mix together well and leave to sit for 20 minutes (while the chicken is cooking).

Serve the chicken scattered with the spring onions and with the salsa on the side.

pictured overleaf

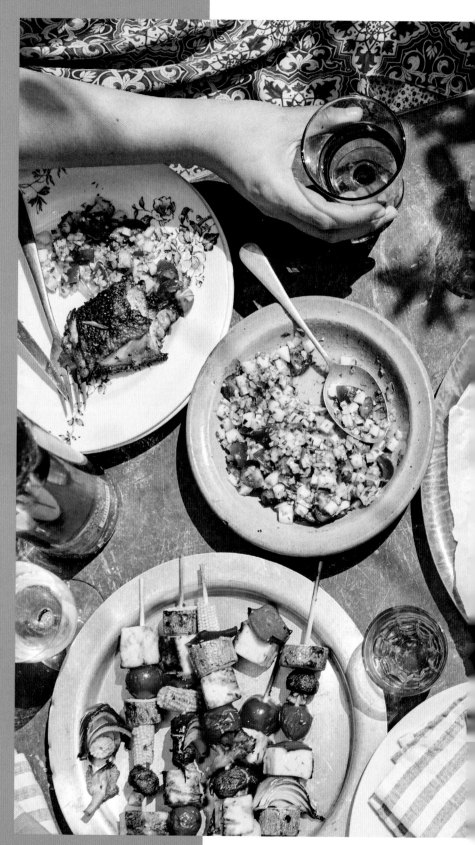

Left to right:
Veg Kebabs Filipino-Style (page 157),
Mango-Tomato Salsa (page 179),
Mum's Filipino Chicken (page 179),
Fried Halloumi Slaw (page 99)

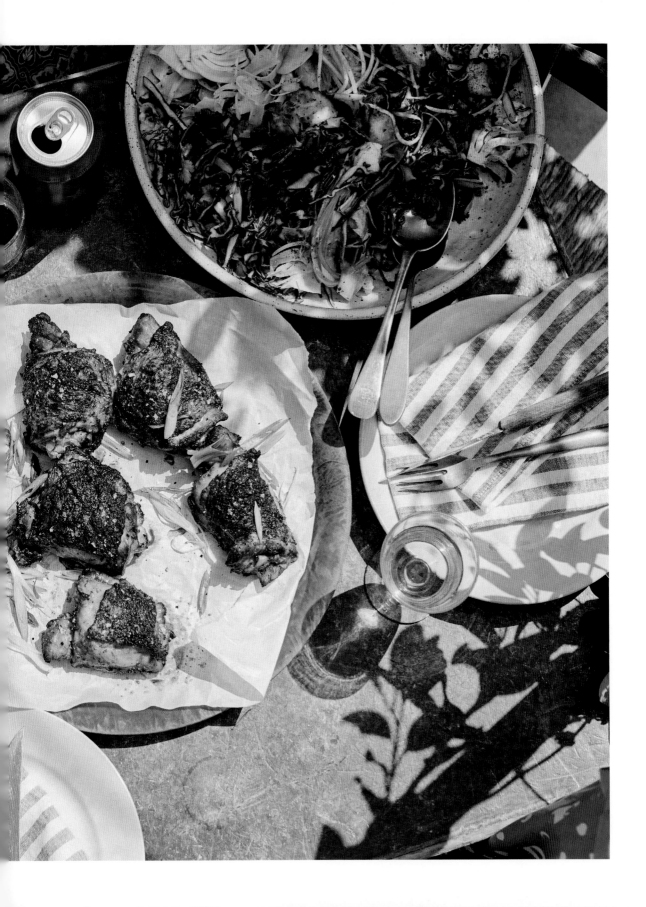

spiced chickpea and fish traybake with garlic yoghurt

feeds 2 ———— 35 minutes

2 tbsp ghee or coconut oil

300g butternut squash, cut into 2cm cubes, skin on

1 large onion, roughly sliced

1 large red pepper, deseeded and roughly chopped

1 large courgette, roughly chopped

400g tin of chickpeas, drained and rinsed

2 fish fillets *(such as trout or wild salmon – 250g in total)*

1 lemon, cut into 4 wedges

Sea salt and black pepper

1 handful of fresh coriander, parsley or dill, roughly chopped, to serve

chermoula-inspired spice mix

1 tbsp cumin seeds or 2 tsp ground cumin

1 tsp smoked paprika

2 tsp ground coriander

A pinch of chilli flakes

garlic yoghurt

3 big garlic cloves, unpeeled

4 tbsp thick natural yoghurt

Veg-packed, colourful and easy as can be in a traybake. The spice mix, inspired by North African chermoula, makes it extra special. I recommend roasting extra garlic cloves when you're making this, and adding them to oils or more dressings and dips – delicious! For veggie friends, I'd add mushrooms to roast instead of fish.

———————————————————————

Preheat the oven to fan 200°C/gas mark 7, then place 1½ tablespoons of the ghee in a large roasting tray and pop in the oven to heat up.

Meanwhile, mix all the ingredients for the chermoula-inspired spice mix in a small bowl with a generous pinch of salt and pepper.

Remove the tray from the oven and add the veg, chickpeas and unpeeled garlic cloves (for the garlic yoghurt), sprinkle over the spice mix and toss in the hot ghee. Spread out in a single, even layer and roast for 20 minutes, tossing after about 12 minutes.

After 20 minutes take out the garlic cloves (which should be softened by now) before tossing everything gently again in the roasting tray. Make two gaps big enough for the fish, then add the fillets (drizzling over the remaining ghee and seasoning with salt and pepper), tuck in the lemon wedges and roast for another 8–10 minutes until the fish is just cooked.

Meanwhile, squeeze the garlic from its skin – use a fork or your hands if the cloves are cool enough to handle – and then mash with a pinch of salt before mixing with the yoghurt in a small bowl.

Once the fish is cooked, serve up the veg (I like to use deep bowls), piling the fish on top, dolloping over the garlic yoghurt and scattering with the herbs to finish. Serve with the roasted lemon wedges to squeeze over the yoghurt and fish.

feel good

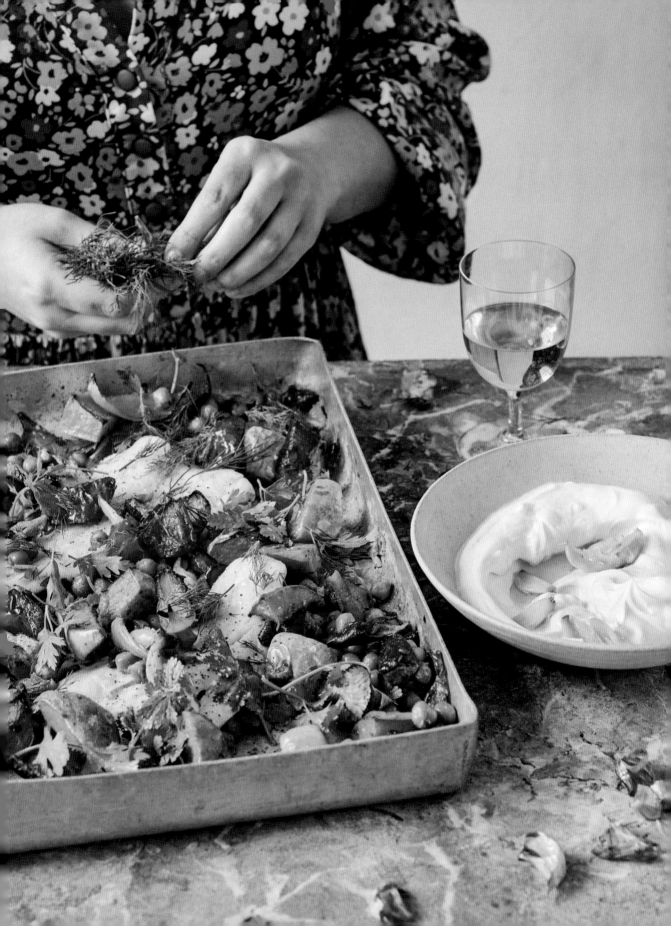

one-tray chicken with ginger-spring-onion salsa

feeds 2 ——— 40 minutes

2 tbsp coconut oil or ghee
2 sweet potatoes, scrubbed and
  sliced into 8mm-thick rounds
2 large chicken thighs, skin on
  and bone in, patted dry
2 tbsp tamari or soy sauce
200g broccoli *(tender-stem
  or regular)*
1½ tsp toasted sesame oil
Sea salt and white pepper

ginger-spring-onion salsa
4 spring onions, green and white
  finely sliced
2 tbsp finely grated fresh ginger
  (from a 5cm piece)
4 tbsp extra-virgin olive oil
2 tsp tamari or soy sauce

to serve
2 lemon or lime wedges
1 handful of chopped coriander
½ small cucumber, thinly sliced
  or peeled into ribbons with
  a vegetable peeler
A pinch of chilli flakes *(optional)*

I love this salsa, which perks up so many dishes. Mix up your veg by swapping in squash, pumpkin or celeriac, and substitute the broccoli with asparagus when in season. The salsa is also delicious on noodles and leftover fried quinoa or rice. Use fish fillets or cubed extra-firm tofu instead of the chicken, if you prefer. The tofu can go in at the same time as the sweet potatoes, but add the fish after the broccoli as it will need only 8–10 minutes in the oven.

Preheat the oven to fan 220°C/gas mark 9, then place the coconut oil in a very large roasting tray and pop in the oven to heat up.

Carefully tumble the sweet potatoes in the hot oil. Add the chicken thighs, sprinkle with a generous pinch of salt and pepper and use tongs or a couple of forks to coat all over in the oil. Drizzle over the tamari or soy sauce and then space out the sweet potatoes in a single layer, sprinkling them with salt and pepper. Nestle the chicken in between the sweet potatoes and roast for 18 minutes.

Meanwhile, mix all the ingredients for the salsa in a small bowl and season to taste with salt and pepper.

Prepare the broccoli by slicing any thicker florets in half lengthways and chopping any thick stems for quicker cooking.

Remove the roasting tray from the oven, gently toss the sweet potatoes and scatter the broccoli around the chicken. Drizzle the broccoli with the toasted sesame oil, season with salt and roast for another 10–12 minutes until the chicken is cooked through and the veg are tender.

Leave the chicken to rest for 5 minutes while you plate up a wedge of lemon or lime, some coriander and a little pile of cucumber slices/ribbons, sprinkled with a little chilli if you like. Pile the sweet potatoes and broccoli next to the cucumber, place the chicken on top and spoon over the salsa to finish.

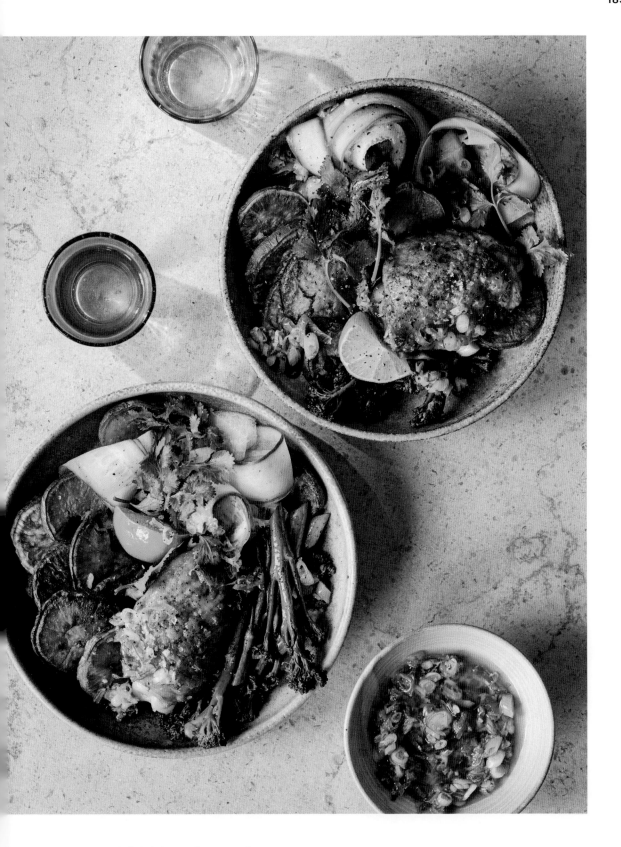

meat and fish (with lots of veg too)

trout, asparagus and potato traybake with garlic-mayo-saffron sauce

feeds 2 ———— 30 minutes

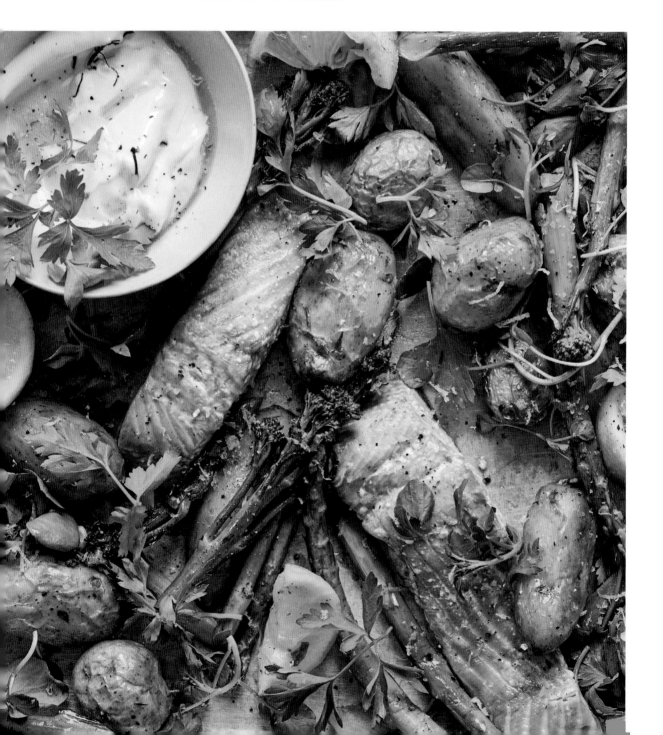

1½ tbsp ghee or oil of your choice

300g potatoes *(see introduction)*, scrubbed and cut into 2.5cm cubes

1 big handful of asparagus spears

2 handfuls of tender-stem broccoli

2 fillets of trout or other fish

½ lemon, sliced into 2 wedges

Sea salt and black pepper

garlic-mayo-saffron sauce

3 saffron strands

2 tbsp good-quality mayonnaise

1 small garlic clove, peeled

to serve

2 big handfuls of watercress, rocket or salad leaves

1 handful of fresh herbs *(such as parsley and dill or mint)*, chopped

A lovely dish to make when asparagus is in season. Out of season, swap the asparagus for green beans. I love this garlic-mayo-saffron sauce as it's looser than mayonnaise, so not too rich. Saffron is expensive but it is oh-so-special and the tiniest amount goes a long way. As an alternative, stir ⅛ teaspoon each of smoked paprika and ground turmeric into your garlic mayo to add a kick of flavour and a great colour. This salad is fantastic with new potatoes, such as Jersey Royals, but use any type of potato that you like.

Preheat the oven to fan 200°C/gas mark 7, then place 1 tablespoon of the ghee in a large roasting tray and pop in the oven to heat up.

Remove the tray from the oven and toss the potatoes in the hot ghee, seasoning with salt and pepper, then spread out in a single layer and roast for 15 minutes.

Meanwhile, prepare the asparagus and broccoli. Snap off the ends of the asparagus spears (saving to use in soups or stocks) and slice any thick pieces of asparagus or broccoli in half lengthways.

Remove the tray from the oven, add the asparagus and broccoli and toss gently with the potatoes, then make two gaps big enough for the trout and add the fillets. Drizzle the remaining ghee over the trout and season with salt and pepper, then tuck in the lemon wedges and roast for about 10 minutes until the fish is just cooked.

Meanwhile, make the sauce. Place the saffron in a small bowl with 2 tablespoons of hot water and leave to soak for 10 minutes before stirring it all into the mayonnaise. Finely chop the garlic, sprinkle with a pinch of salt and use the back of your knife or a spoon to smoosh and smash the garlic into a paste before stirring this through the sauce.

Once the trout is cooked, divide the watercress or other leaves between two plates, serve up the fish and veg, spoon over the sauce, scatter over the herbs and squeeze over the roasted lemon wedges to finish.

meat and fish (with lots of veg too)

quick Cambodian-style fish curry

feeds 2 ———— 30 minutes

2 tsp coconut oil or ghee
10 cherry tomatoes
400ml tin of coconut milk
250g firm white fish fillets
10 asparagus spears
2 handfuls of baby spinach
Sea salt and black pepper

yellow curry paste

2 lemongrass stalks, outer leaves
　discarded and inner part
　roughly chopped or 2 tsp paste
2 garlic cloves, peeled
1 medium onion or 2 shallots,
　roughly chopped
Juice of ½ lime and grated zest,
　or 2 Makrut lime leaves
2 tsp grated fresh ginger or
　1 tsp finely sliced galangal
½ tsp ground turmeric
2 tsp fish sauce
½ tsp *(coconut)* sugar or maple
　syrup
A pinch of chilli flakes

to serve

½ lime, cut into 2 wedges
2 handfuls of fresh herbs
　(such as coriander, basil or mint),
　roughly chopped

variation

For a plant-based version,
roast 1 aubergine, cut into
chunks, and add instead
of the fish. Use a vegan fish
sauce in the curry paste.

Based on fish *amok*, one of Cambodia's national dishes, this is made a using a homemade yellow curry paste or *kroeung*. It isn't a spicy curry, but feel free to add as much chilli as you like. Use green beans if asparagus isn't in season. If you find it tricky to get lemongrass, buy extra when you can and freeze it (which is what I do!); it defrosts quickly. This is great served with a side of quinoa, noodles or griddled wraps.

Place all the ingredients for the yellow curry paste in a food processor and blitz into a fairly smooth paste. Add a tablespoon or two of water to get it going, if needed, and pulse a few times. Alternatively, pound the solid ingredients together using a pestle and mortar before mixing with the ground and liquid ingredients.

Melt the coconut oil in a medium frying pan, add the curry paste and cook on a medium heat for 3 minutes, stirring regularly to prevent it from catching. Add the cherry tomatoes and a pinch of salt, stir to coat in the paste and then fry for another minute.

Stir in the coconut milk, turn up the heat and cook on a medium simmer for 10 minutes to let the sauce reduce slightly and thicken.

Pat the fish dry, cut into 2.5cm cubes, and sprinkle over a little salt and pepper.

Prepare the asparagus by snapping off the woody ends, then roughly chop the asparagus stems so that they cook quickly and are easier to eat.

Add the fish and asparagus to the curry, spacing them out in the sauce, and gently poach for about 5 minutes with a lid on the pan, then scatter the spinach among the fish and asparagus, pop the lid back on and cook for another 3–4 minutes until the fish is cooked through. Take off the heat, pushing the wilted spinach into the sauce, then taste the curry and adjust the seasoning if needed.

Serve straight away with lime wedges and pile high with herbs.

feel good

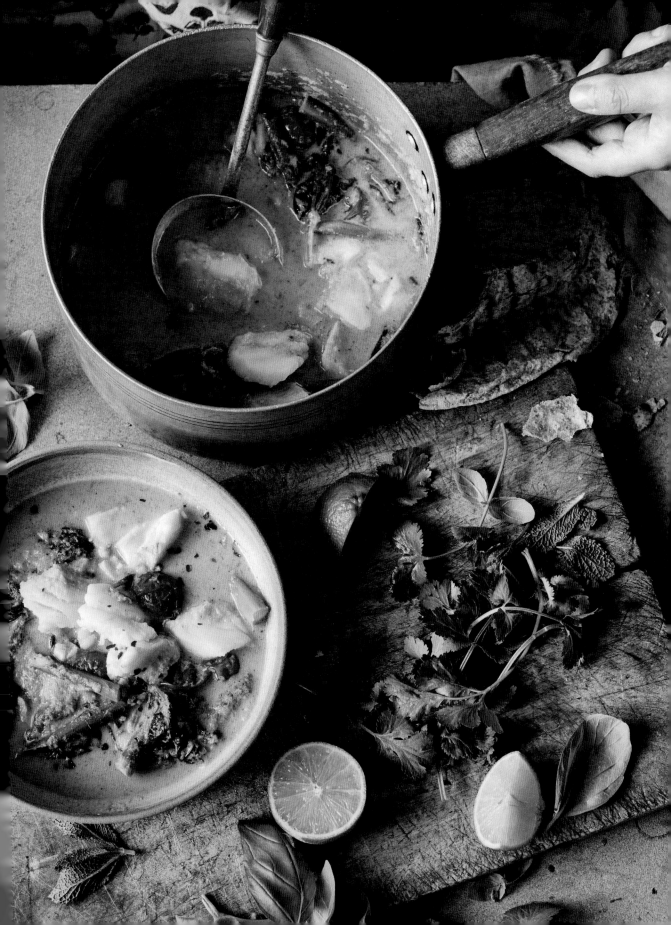

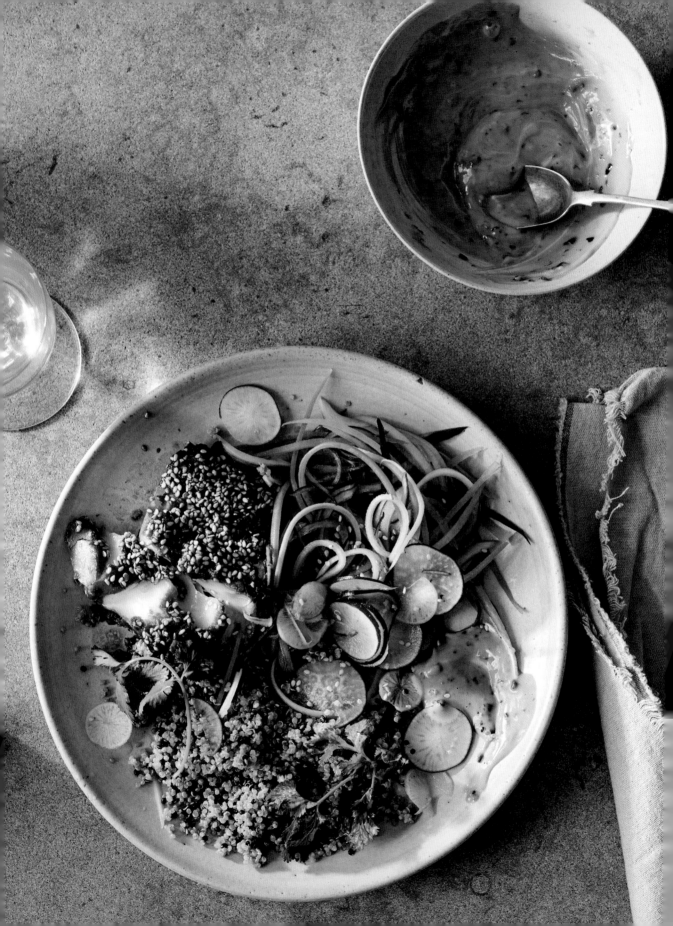

sesame fish with tricolour quinoa

feeds 2 ——— 30 minutes

2 fish fillets, skin on

140g tricolour quinoa, rinsed

Ghee or coconut oil, for greasing

1 handful of black and white
sesame seeds, plus extra to serve

1 handful of fresh coriander,
roughly chopped

Sea salt

sauce

3 tbsp tamari or soy sauce

1 tbsp toasted sesame oil

1 garlic clove, finely chopped

2 tsp chilli sauce or a pinch of
chilli flakes *(or to taste)*

2 tsp maple syrup

to serve

Quick-pickled Veg *(page 246)*

Spicy Mayo *(page 246)*

Use wild fish fillets, if you can, from a sustainable source. I've used tricolour quinoa here (a mixture of white, red and black) for added texture, colour and nuttiness, but use regular quinoa instead, if you like, which takes a little less time to cook. Wild rice would work well too, though it takes almost twice as long as the quinoa to cook. The **Spicy Mayo** (page 246) is perfect alongside this, and is very quick to make as it uses many of the same ingredients as in the sauce.

Mix the sauce ingredients together in a wide bowl. Place the fish, flesh side down, in the sauce and let it sit for 15 minutes while you get on with everything else.

Cook the quinoa in a medium saucepan (according to the packet instructions – usually around 18 minutes or 15 minutes for regular quinoa) in about 300ml of water with a pinch of sea salt and with a lid on the pan. Remove from the hob and leave for 4 minutes off the heat before taking off the lid and fluffing the quinoa with a fork.

Preheat the grill to high and then place the fish, skin side down, on a greased baking tray, drizzle over any remaining sauce and sprinkle over the sesame seeds. Grill for 6–8 minutes until the fish is just cooked through (it will carry on cooking when removed from the heat).

While the fish is cooking, divide the **Quick-pickled Veg** between two plates and top with the fresh coriander. Transfer the hot quinoa and fish to the plates with a spoonful of **Spicy Mayo**.

one-pan oregano chicken and chickpeas

feeds 4 ———— 50 minutes

1 tsp smoked paprika
A pinch of chilli flakes
2 tsp dried oregano
4 large chicken thighs, skin on
  and bone in
2 tbsp ghee or olive oil
1 large onion, finely diced
1 large carrot, finely diced
2 red peppers, deseeded and
  diced into 1cm cubes
4 garlic cloves, finely chopped
2 tbsp tomato purée
300ml veg or chicken stock
400g tin of chopped tomatoes
400g tin of chickpeas, drained
  and rinsed
200g quinoa or rice, rinsed well
2 handfuls of *(black)* pitted olives
Sea salt and black pepper

to serve
Juice of ½ lemon and a little
  grated zest and remaining
  ½ lemon cut into 4 wedges
2 handfuls of parsley, finely
  chopped
150g feta, crumbled

This is lovely served with a big salad of lettuce, cucumber and chicory leaves dressed in lemon juice and olive oil. I prefer to buy chicken thighs with the skin on and bone in, as the meat is juicier and easier to not overcook. You could swap chicken for a firm white fish that you'd press in the rub ingredients, as in the first step, and then add in the final 5 minutes of the quinoa cooking time. This is also great with rice. Check out my veg variation on the next page.

Scatter the smoked paprika and chilli flakes on a plate or in a bowl, along with a good pinch of salt and pepper and 1 teaspoon of the dried oregano. Press the chicken, skin side down, into the mixture, then turn over and press the other side into the mix.

Heat up 1 tablespoon of the ghee in a large pan with a lid, then add the chicken, skin side down, and cook on a medium–high heat for 6–8 minutes until nicely golden brown on that side, then, once the chicken comes away easily from the pan, turn and cook the other side for another 2–3 minutes. (Tongs really help here.) Transfer the chicken to a clean plate and set aside.

Add the remaining ghee to the pan, if needed (the chicken will have released some fat during cooking so you may not have to add any extra ghee), tip in the onion and fry on a medium heat for 5 minutes, stirring from time to time, then add the rest of the veg and cook for another 5 minutes, stirring occasionally, before adding the garlic to cook for a final minute.

Make a gap in the mix, stir in the tomato purée and stir-fry for a minute in the gap before stirring into the other ingredients in the pan. Stir in the stock, scraping the bottom of the pan as you mix it in, and then add the tinned tomatoes, chickpeas, quinoa and a pinch of salt and pepper. Stir everything together well, especially at the bottom of the pan, then pop the lid on and bring to a strong simmer.

continued overleaf

feel good

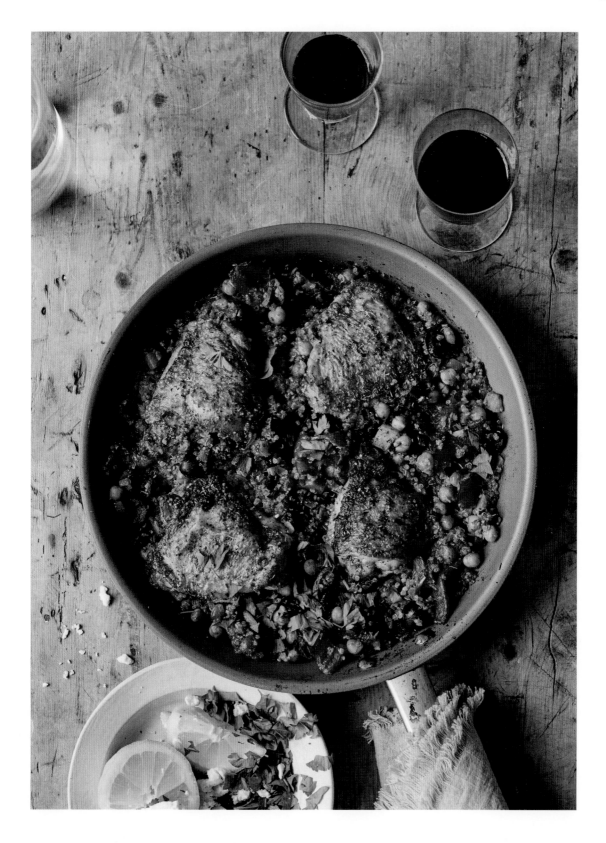

meat and fish (with lots of veg too)

Straight away remove the lid, stir again and, using tongs, place the chicken, skin side up, in the pan, replace the lid and simmer on a medium-low heat for 18–20 minutes until the quinoa is tender and the chicken is cooked through. Halfway through the cooking time, stir the quinoa thoroughly but gently, scraping the bottom of the pan once again to make sure the quinoa doesn't stick (if it helps, remove the chicken, give the quinoa a stir and then pop the chicken back in). If you feel the quinoa needs a bit more liquid, pour in 100ml of hot water (about half a mug), drizzling it around the quinoa. Having stirred the quinoa, scatter the olives around the chicken before leaving to cook for the remaining time.

Remove the pan from the heat, take off the lid and leave to sit for 5 minutes.

To finish, stir the lemon juice and zest, half the herbs and half the feta into the quinoa, fluff the quinoa a bit with a fork and taste for seasoning. Serve with the lemon wedges and scattered with the rest of the herbs and feta.

variations

This recipe is Greek-inspired; for an Italian-style variation, swap the feta for Parmesan and add fresh basil with the parsley.

For a veggie version, use 400g roughly chopped mixed mushrooms and brown them as you would the chicken before setting aside and adding at the end. I'd also add deli-style artichoke hearts.

tip

If you have leftover cooked quinoa and feta, once cold, add a whisked egg and a few tablespoons of flour, season to taste and form into fritters. Fry gently until golden brown, then flip and fry the other side.

sweet potato fishcakes and simple salad

feeds 4, makes 12 medium fishcakes ———— 50 minutes

2 tbsp ghee or coconut oil,
plus extra for frying

600g sweet potatoes or potatoes,
scrubbed and chopped into
2cm chunks

400g skinless and boneless fish
fillets *(about 3 medium fillets)*

100g frozen peas

2 eggs

1–2 tsp strong mustard *(to taste)*

3 spring onions or ½ small onion,
finely chopped

1 handful of parsley, finely chopped

1 tbsp capers, roughly chopped

Juice of ½ lemon and a little
grated zest

3–4 tbsp flour *(plain, buckwheat
or chickpea/gram)*, plus extra
for shaping the fishcakes

Sea salt and black pepper

simple salad

Leaves from 4 Little Gem lettuces

½ cucumber, finely sliced

1 small handful of fresh mint
leaves or dill

tartare-style dressing

4 tbsp extra-virgin olive oil

Juice of ½ lemon

2 tbsp natural yoghurt

3 tbsp chopped cornichons,
gherkins or capers

This is more of a hands-on recipe, but I adore these fishcakes and they're worth it! The extra veg means a conservative amount of fish goes a long way. If you have left overs, they are delicious the next day, and they freeze well. Use different types of fish, but go for a firm white variety or wild salmon – whatever the fishmonger says is sustainable and responsibly sourced. The salad with tartare-style dressing gives a fresh and tangy contrast to the fishcakes. I like to keep the peel on the potatoes but if you'd rather have neater fishcakes, peel them.

Preheat the oven to fan 190°C/gas mark 6½, then place the ghee in a large roasting tray and pop in the oven to heat up.

Add the sweet potatoes (or potatoes) to the tray, season with a good pinch of salt and pepper and carefully toss in the melted ghee, then spread out in a single layer and roast for 15 minutes.

Pull the tray out, toss the sweet potatoes, then move a little to one side to make space and add the fish fillets to the empty side of the tray. Sprinkle with salt and pepper and pop back in the oven to bake for another 8 minutes until the fish is just cooked and the sweet potatoes are tender. Remove the tray from the oven but keep the oven on low so the fishcakes can be kept warm later.

Meanwhile, cover the frozen peas with boiling water in a small bowl. In a medium mixing bowl, whisk the eggs with a fork. Add the mustard, if using, a generous pinch of salt and pepper, and the spring onions/onion, parsley, capers, lemon juice and zest and peas, once drained.

Use a fork or potato masher to mash the sweet potatoes in the roasting tray, avoiding the fish. This will help the sweet potatoes to cool down more quickly so that the fishcakes stick together when you are frying them.

continued overleaf

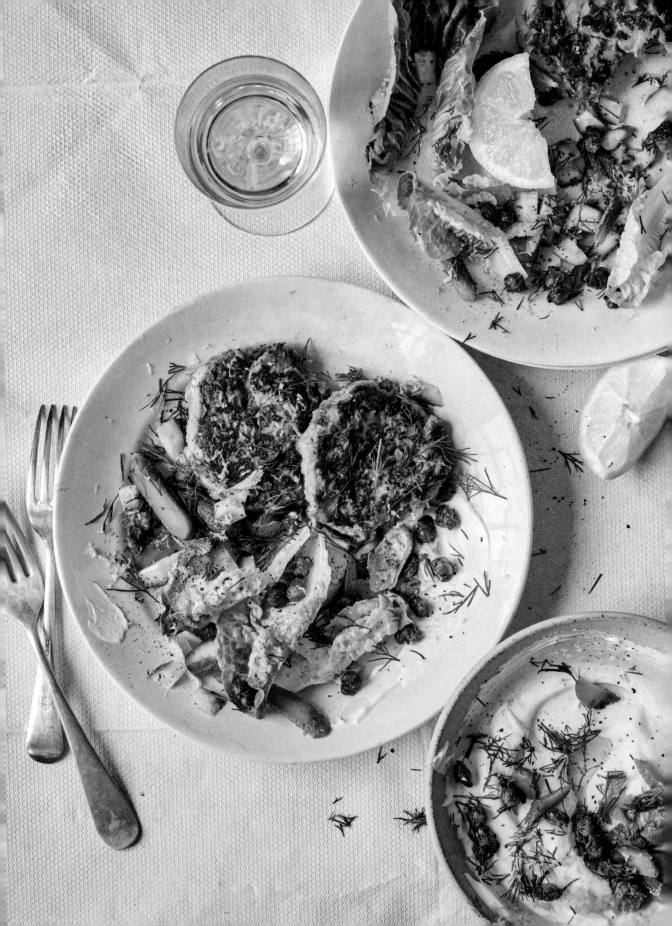

Add the mashed sweet potatoes and 2–3 tablespoons of flour to the mixing bowl, then combine with the other ingredients before roughly flaking in the fish and gently mixing in. Taste for seasoning. If you have time, pop the bowl into the fridge to chill and firm up for 20 minutes, but don't worry if not.

Using floured hands, form the fishcake mixture into 12 even-sized patties. If they feel wet when shaping, add another 1 tablespoon flour. Fry them in batches, spaced out in a large frying pan on a medium–high heat in a spoonful of melted ghee. Be sure to not overcrowd the pan (hence frying in batches), or they will steam rather than crisp up. Cook on one side for 3 minutes, undisturbed, then gently turn and fry on the other side for another 2 minutes or so. As all the ingredients are cooked already, you're just warming them through and getting a nice golden finish on each side. Keep any cooked fishcakes warm in the roasting tray in the oven and, between batches, remove any leftover bits in the pan or they will burn, and add a little more ghee to make sure the next batch of fishcakes doesn't stick.

To make the salad, mix the ingredients for the dressing in a serving platter (you can do this in advance), then just before eating, add the salad leaves, cucumber and fresh herbs and toss together.

tip

If you want to prep ahead, shape the fishcakes and keep them in the fridge, then bring them out 30 minutes before cooking.

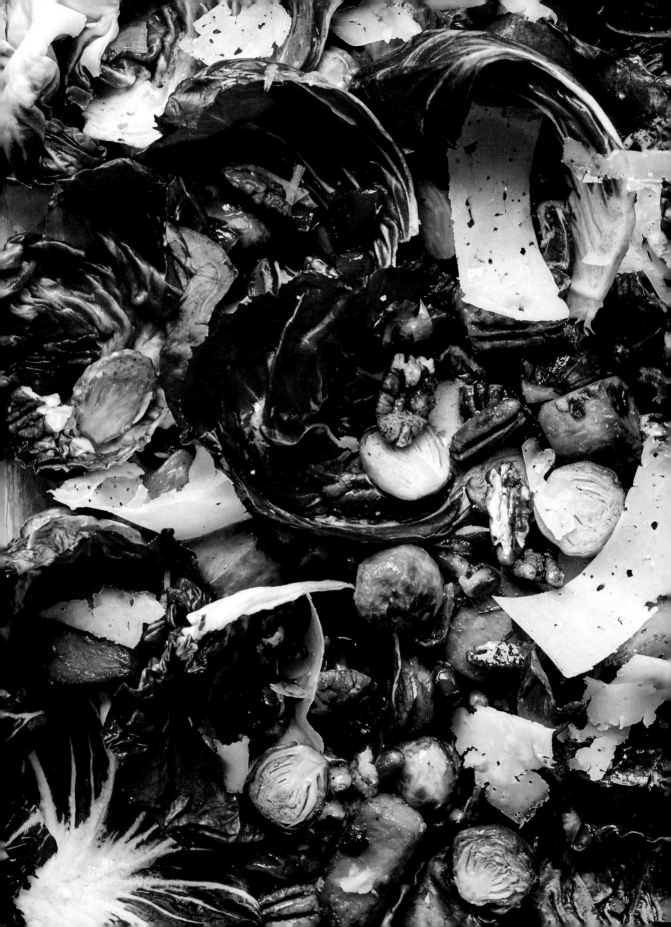

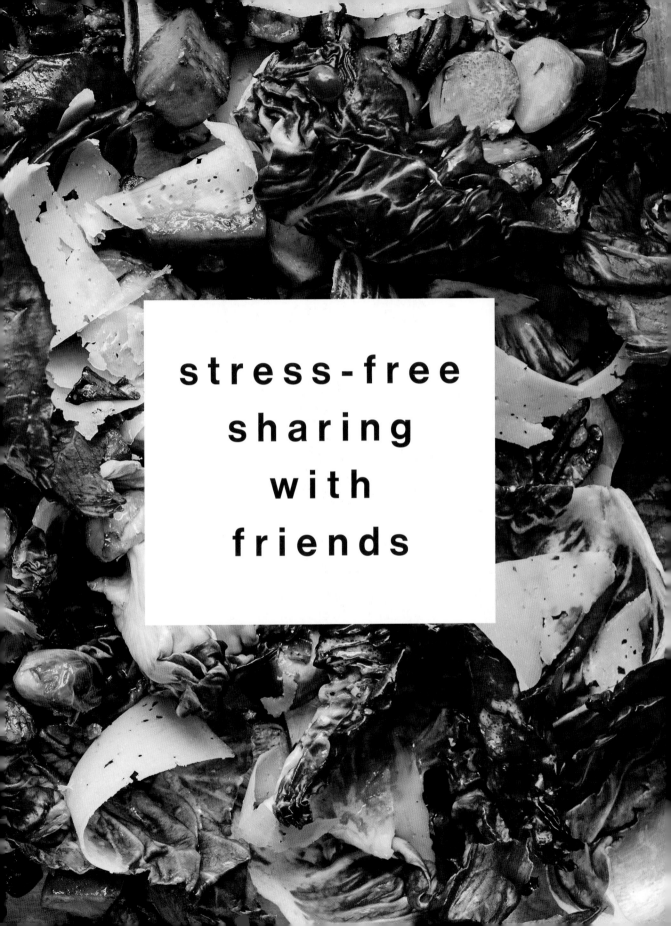

stress-free
sharing
with
friends

/ these recipes are really simple to whip up /

I made a promise to myself years ago to only invite people round if I wasn't going to get stressed. So, these recipes are either really simple to whip up, even if your guests have arrived and you're still busy multitasking to get everything done, or they can be prepared in the morning to ensure your evening of entertaining is frazzle-free and, as it should be, a pleasure.

There are so many recipes in the book that work well for sharing, whether as a selection of smaller dishes, or a big batch of something hot and filling with a fresh salad, salsa or slaw on the side, letting everyone help themselves. For ease and visual impact, I love making up party platters (sharing boards) as they are the ultimate in 'graze and laze' and very convivial. There'll be something on there for everyone and if you're in a rush, you can supplement with a few shop-bought, ready-made things too. You'll find a veggie-loaded platter (page 214) that includes **Sweet Potato Rounds and Roasted Chickpeas** to enjoy with a **Whipped Feta Dip Swirled with Harissa Honey** and lots of other delicious extras to go with it.

I must give a special mention to the **Farinata** (page 218), which is one of my favourite recipes in the whole book. A full-flavoured, crispy chickpea pancake, made with plenty of olive oil, it's both rich and light and absolutely delicious. It takes just 10 minutes of hands-on time and you can switch up the toppings according to what you have in the cupboard or fridge. Please make it – you'll love it!

If you're going to a friend's house for a barbecue or want to make a contribution to a picnic, I'd highly recommend the **Charred Corn and Avocado Salad** (page 100). Or, even better, bring a few of the wonderfully easy **Three-Ingredient Chocolate Pots** (page 230) with you too.

In other chapters, look out for:

- **Aubergine Skewers with Cucumber Ribbons** (page 141)
- **Mushroom and Aubergine Pancakes with Sesame Sauce** (page 158)
- **Loaded Root Veg Wedges with *Mojo Verde* and Tahini Yoghurt** (page 166)

black bean and sweet potato wraps with chipotle mayo

feeds 4 ——— 30 minutes

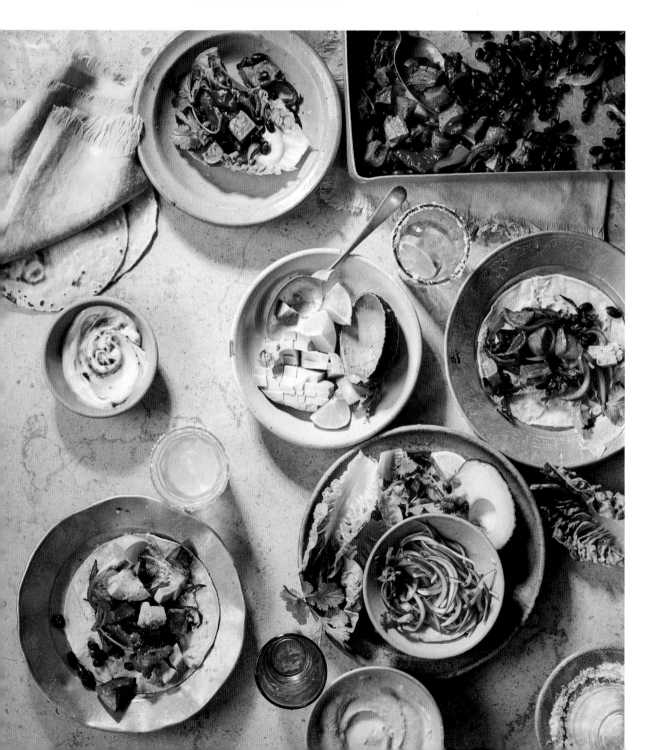

8 wraps (*see introduction*) and
leaves of 2 Little Gem lettuces

filling
3 tbsp ghee or coconut oil
400g tin of black beans,
drained and rinsed
1 large (*red*) onion, roughly sliced
2 large sweet potatoes, scrubbed
and cut into 2cm cubes
2 large red peppers, deseeded
and roughly chopped
½ tsp chilli flakes (*look out for
chipotle chilli*)
2 tsp ground cumin
2 tsp smoked paprika
1 ½ tsp dried oregano
Sea salt and black pepper

coriander-lime drizzle
6 tbsp Greek-style yoghurt or
dairy-free alternative
1 garlic clove
2 handfuls of fresh coriander,
saving a few leaves for garnishing
½–1 fresh jalapeño or other
(*green*) chilli (*to taste*), deseeded
if you prefer
Juice of 1 lime and grated zest

chipotle mayo
3 tbsp mayonnaise or
Greek-style yoghurt
1 tbsp chipotle paste, or use
hot sauce or harissa paste

optional extras
Sliced red onion, or pickled
onion (*page 246*)
Sliced ripe avocado, or Mango-
Tomato Salsa (*page 179*)
Crumbled feta or grated
Cheddar (*or use queso fresco
or Cotija, if you can get it*)

There are so many ways to serve this: as wraps, like I've done here, or as a DIY bowl, mixed with some cooked quinoa or rice. Or fold your filled wraps and toast both sides in a pan, then slice them up. For the wraps, I like to use a mixture of toasted or warmed corn tortillas or chickpea wraps and crunchy lettuce boats.

Preheat the oven to fan 220°C/gas mark 9, then place the ghee in two large roasting trays and pop in the oven to heat up.

Dry the rinsed beans in a clean tea towel so that they roast rather than steam and don't spit in the hot oil.

Once the ghee has melted, tumble the onion, veg and beans into the roasting trays, evenly spread to avoid overcrowding, and scatter over the spices, oregano and a pinch of salt and pepper. Toss together and spread out in a single, even layer, then roast for 15 minutes. Remove the trays from the oven, toss again and roast for another 10 minutes until the sweet potato is tender and going golden at the edges.

While the veg are roasting, pop all the ingredients for the coriander-lime drizzle into a food processor or blender and blitz until smooth, then season with salt and pepper to taste and pour into a small bowl so everyone can help themselves. Alternatively, just chop all the solid ingredients and mix in a small bowl with the yoghurt and lime juice and zest.

Mix the chipotle mayo ingredients together in another small bowl with 1 tablespoon of water and season to taste with salt.

Place any optional extras on a large platter and make sure any lettuce leaves (for using as wraps) are nice and dry. Around 5 minutes before the roasted veg are ready, pop any wraps that need warming into a dry frying pan to toast on each side, then wrap them in a clean tea towel to keep them warm and to stop them drying out. You could warm them in the oven instead, but I think they taste best when they are dry-fried in a pan.

Serve up and let everyone DIY their wraps, helping themselves to the roasted beans and veg, coriander-lime drizzle, chipotle mayo and any extras.

courgette-feta fritters with chive yoghurt

makes 12 fritters ——— 45 minutes

600g courgettes
½ onion or 4 spring onions,
   finely chopped
2 eggs
1 lemon
60g ground almonds, plus extra
   if needed
1 handful of herbs *(such as parsley,*
   mint or dill), finely chopped
½ tsp ground cumin or smoked
   paprika or a little pinch of chilli
   flakes *(optional)*
80g feta, crumbled
2 tbsp ghee or olive oil, for frying
Sea salt and black pepper

chive yoghurt

200g Greek-style yoghurt
1 small garlic clove, finely grated
   or chopped
2 tbsp finely chopped chives or
   1 finely chopped spring onion

to serve

Chopped tomatoes sprinkled with
   dried oregano and a little salt
   and pepper

I make fritters regularly, often on a Friday ('Friday Fritters'!), as they are a fantastic way of using up veg that needs eating. See also my **Sweetcorn-Carrot Fritters** (page 146). They are so versatile: serve them hot, crispy and bite-sized as canapés or a starter, or pile them high on a party platter. You could make them the night before a road trip for a travel snack as they are also delicious cold. The chive yoghurt makes a lovely tangy contrast to the fritters. Go for smaller courgettes, if you can, as they tend to be less watery.

Grate the courgettes using the coarse side of a box grater, then transfer to a bowl, sprinkle with a little salt and mix in well. Leave for 15 minutes while you get on with everything else.

Whisk the eggs in a second bowl and use the fine side of the box grater to grate in a little lemon zest, avoiding the bitter white pith, then cut the lemon into wedges for serving later. Add the ground almonds, chopped herbs, spices (if using) and some salt and pepper.

For the yoghurt, mix everything together in a small bowl, season to taste with salt and pepper and set aside.

Place the salted courgettes in a clean tea towel, squeeze well and discard the excess juice. You don't need to get rid of all the moisture, just the excess, as you don't want dry fritters. Add the squeezed courgettes to the bowl with the eggs and chopped onion or spring onions. Mix well with your hands and then add the crumbled feta and combine. If the mixture is too wet, add 1 tablespoon more of the ground almonds; if too dry, whisk an extra egg in a small bowl and add as much as needed to the mixture.

continued overleaf

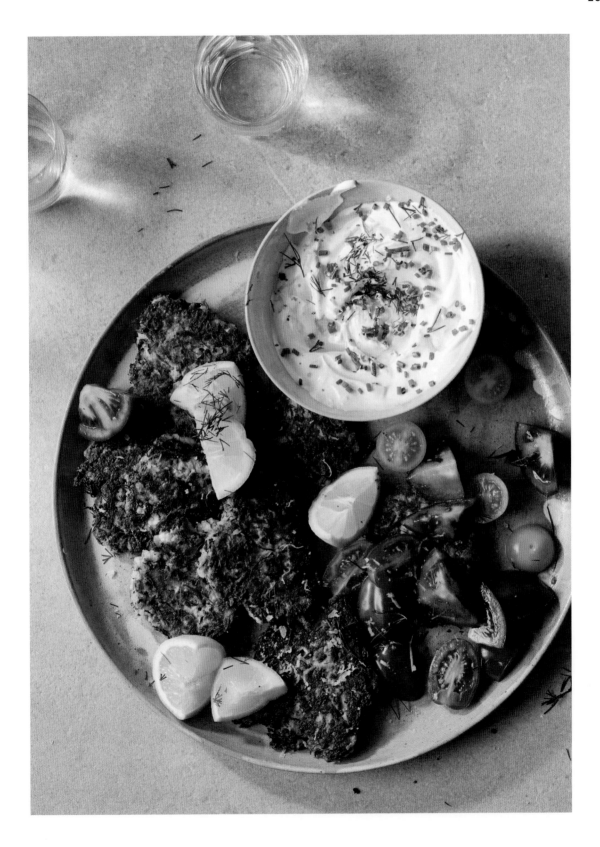

stress-free sharing with friends

Place a large frying pan on a medium-high heat and heat up 2 teaspoons of the ghee, making sure it covers the base of the pan. Add about 2 tablespoons of batter per fritter to the pan – and add as many fritters as you can while keeping them spaced apart and not overcrowding the pan (I manage to fit six fritters in my frying pan). Use a spatula to press down slightly to gently flatten them a little, then cook for 3 minutes before carefully flipping and cooking the other side for another 2 minutes or so until golden all over – they'll be crispy on the outside and still a bit soft inside. Transfer them to a large plate – again, spaced apart rather than too crowded together or they might steam and lose their crispiness. Pop into the oven on a low heat to keep hot, if you like, though I quite like them served warm.

Between batches, scrape out any bits from the pan or they may burn, add 2 teaspoons more ghee and repeat until you have 12 fritters. Enjoy straight away with the yoghurt, lemon wedges and tomato salad.

tip

Double the recipe and freeze leftover cooked fritters. Defrost and bake in the oven at fan 190°C/gas mark 6½ for about 15 minutes until hot and crisp at the edges.

grilled marinated peppers with herbs, capers and olives

makes 1 big jar ———— 1 hour *(hands-on time 20 minutes)*

6 large peppers *(red, orange and yellow)*
2 garlic cloves, finely sliced
2 tbsp capers
2 tbsp pitted olives
1 tsp dried oregano or 1 tbsp chopped fresh oregano or thyme leaves
8 tbsp extra-virgin olive oil
3 tbsp balsamic vinegar
2 tsp maple syrup
Sea salt and black pepper

optional extras
1 handful of toasted chopped almonds or pine nuts, to serve
1 handful of crumbled feta or mozzarella or Parmesan shavings, to serve

A super-versatile staple. In the summer months, I make a big jar of these once a week to add to salads. They are especially good tossed with some cooked lentils or mixed beans, or on top of flatbreads and pizzas. They are perfect for preparing ahead for a party as they taste even better after marinating overnight. I have an induction hob, so my method is to cook them under the grill or in the oven, but if you've got a barbecue or gas hob, you could char them instead.

Preheat the grill to high or the oven to fan 200°C/gas mark 7.

Pop the whole peppers on a large baking sheet. If using the grill, grill for 25 minutes, using tongs to turn them every 8 minutes or so. If using the oven, roast for 35 minutes turning the peppers halfway through the cooking time. You want the pepper skins to blister all over and blacken.

Place the peppers on a chopping board and cover with a large bowl, or pop them in a large bowl and cover with a plate. Leave them to steam for about 20 minutes, then peel the skin off each pepper, remove the seeds and discard.

Meanwhile, add all the other ingredients to an airtight container or large clean jar with a lid and taste for seasoning.

Slice the peppers lengthways about 2cm thick and add them to your container or jar, then stir or shake well to combine. Leave, covered, in the fridge overnight, if you can, or make them in the morning so they have time to marinate before you enjoy them. Scatter over the optional extras to serve.

friendsgiving salad

feeds 6 as a side ———— 35 minutes

2½ tbsp ghee or coconut oil
1 large red onion, roughly
  chopped
2 handfuls of Brussels sprouts,
  halved, or cauliflower florets
700g sweet potatoes *(about 2
  medium)*, scrubbed, or squash
  (see tip), cut into 2.5cm cubes
2 tsp dried thyme or mixed herbs
Sea salt and black pepper

sticky pecans
1 handful of pecans *(or walnuts)*
1 tbsp maple syrup

dressing
3 tbsp extra-virgin olive oil
1½ tbsp apple cider vinegar
½ tsp maple syrup
1 tsp Dijon mustard
1 small garlic clove, finely
  chopped

to serve
1 head of radicchio, sliced, or
  1 big handful of salad leaves
1 handful of pomegranate seeds
  or dried cranberries or 1 small
  chopped apple
1 handful of cheese shavings
  *(such as pecorino, Manchego or
  Parmesan – use a veg peeler)*

tip

Save the seeds from your
squash. Simply clean, dry and
roast with a little sea salt and oil
for a 'no waste' snack.

This is inspired by the big 'holiday' salads served at Thanksgiving celebrations in America. I find a big platter like this so cheerful and fun to share as part of feast. It's got all those beautiful colourful autumnal vegetables and sweet and salty flavours. I feel there's been a growing love of sprouts in recent years, but if you still can't stand them (!), swap them for cauliflower. To make this heartier and to feed four as a main meal, cook up 200g quinoa or lentils, double the dressing and gently toss together to serve.

Preheat the oven to fan 220°C/gas mark 9, then place the ghee in a very large roasting tray and pop in the oven to heat up.

Take the hot tray out of the oven and tumble the veg into the tray with the dried herbs and a generous pinch of salt and pepper. Gently toss together in the hot ghee, spread out on the tray in a single layer and roast for about 25 minutes, tossing halfway through. Take out of the oven when the veg are tender but not too soft (check with a knife) and going golden at the edges.

Roughly break the pecans or walnuts apart in your hands as you scatter them over a medium frying pan and toast on a medium heat for 2–3 minutes, shaking the pan halfway through the cooking time. Drizzle over the maple syrup and a pinch of salt, stir into the nuts and cook for another 30 seconds before taking straight off the heat and leaving to cool.

Place all the ingredients for the dressing in a bowl or clean jar with a lid, season to taste with salt and pepper and stir or shake well.

Tumble the roast veg onto a serving platter and gently toss with the dressing and the radicchio or salad leaves. Scatter over the sticky nuts, fresh pomegranate seeds and cheese shavings to finish.

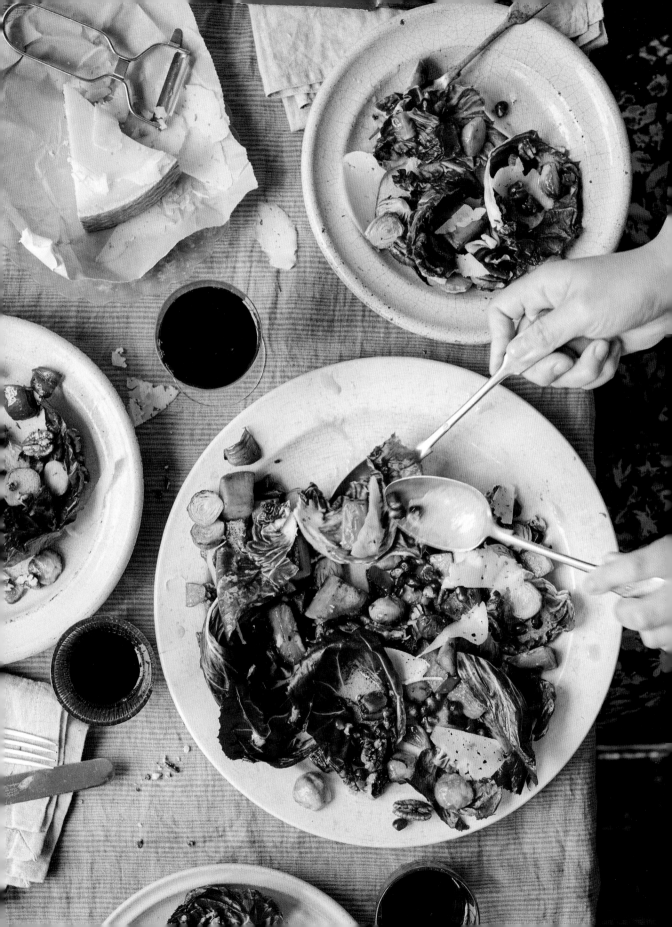

fish finger tacos with avocado cream

feeds 2 ——— 30 minutes

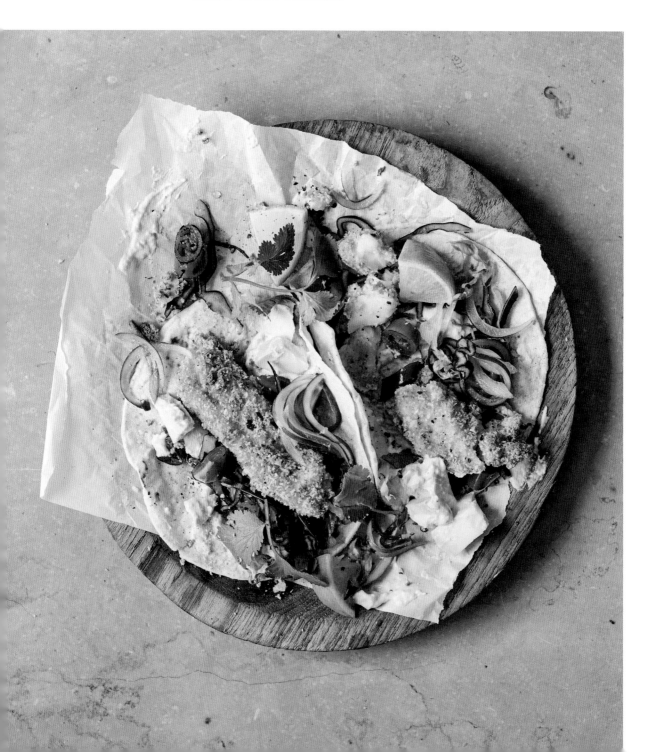

Ghee or olive oil, for greasing
250g firm white skinless fish
  fillets *(see introduction)*
1 egg
80g ground almonds
½ tsp ground cumin
½ tsp smoked paprika
A pinch of *(chipotle)* chilli flakes
1 garlic clove, finely grated
  or chopped
1 tsp grated lime zest
Sea salt and black pepper

slaw
4 handfuls of finely sliced *(red)*
  cabbage and lettuce
2 handfuls of fresh coriander,
  chopped
A few shakes of hot sauce or
  a chopped pickled jalapeño
1 tbsp extra-virgin olive oil
2 tsp lime juice

avocado cream
1 small ripe avocado, peeled
  and pitted
3 tbsp Greek-style yoghurt
  or sour cream
1 ½ tbsp lime juice

to serve
4–6 small corn tortillas
  or other wraps
Sliced red onion or pickled
  onion *(page 246)*
2 lime wedges

The breadcrumb-esque crust of ground almonds works well here but, for a variation, try a mixture of almonds and desiccated coconut or grated Parmesan, if you like. Use a fish such as coley, pollock, haddock, cod or sea bream, or whatever is currently sustainably/ responsibly sourced – ask your fishmonger for up-to-date advice.

Preheat the oven to fan 210°C/gas mark 8 and grease a baking tray or line it with baking parchment.

Pat the fish dry, then slice into 8–10 fingers and season with salt and pepper. Whisk the egg in a small bowl with a little salt and pepper, then mix the ground almonds in another bowl with the spices, half of the garlic and lime zest.

Dip each fish finger into the beaten egg and then in the ground almond mix, ensuring that they are fully coated before placing on the prepared baking tray. Bake on the top shelf of the oven for 15 minutes until cooked through and golden brown.

While the fish is cooking, make the slaw by mixing everything together in a serving bowl with a pinch of salt and pepper.

Next, make the avocado cream. Mash the avocado in another serving bowl with a fork, then add the rest of the ingredients plus the reserved garlic, season generously with salt and pepper and mix together well. It should be creamy and tangy.

Some tortillas are best warmed in the oven (check the packet instructions) but most, I think, are tastiest heated on both sides in a dry pan until lightly golden and charred. Only heat them just before the fish is ready and keep them warm wrapped in a clean tea towel.

Serve up the fish fingers with the slaw, avocado cream, wraps (still in their tea towel to keep warm), sliced red onion and lime wedges and let everyone assemble the tacos themselves.

tomatoes two ways
with burrata

feeds 4 as a side ———— 40 minutes

6 medium ripe tomatoes, halved
1 tbsp olive oil or melted ghee
   or butter
1 tbsp dried rosemary or
   thyme or 2 tsp chopped
   fresh herb leaves
2 burrata
2 handfuls of ripe cherry
   tomatoes, halved
4 tbsp extra-virgin olive oil
1 tbsp pomegranate molasses
   or a few tsp thick balsamic
   vinegar
1 handful of fresh basil leaves
   and a few fresh mint leaves
Sea salt and black pepper

For special occasions, extra-creamy soft burrata is a real treat, though you could swap for mozzarella here, if you prefer. I made this salad with my friend Fiona one hot summer's day for lunch round at hers. She used homegrown vine tomatoes, cherry tomatoes and fresh herbs, with her little boy helping to pick. The key here is tasty, good-quality ingredients and making sure the burrata is room temperature, not cold, so you can really enjoy the flavours.

———————————————————————

Preheat the oven to fan 210°C/gas mark 8.

Lay the halved bigger tomatoes on a baking tray, cut side up and spaced apart, drizzle with the olive oil, sprinkle with the herbs and a little salt and pepper and roast for about 30 minutes until golden at the edges.

Meanwhile, take the burrata out of the fridge so it can come to room temperature, drain it of the excess liquid and then place it on a serving dish.

Once the tomatoes are roasted, arrange them on the serving dish with the burrata and dot the raw cherry tomatoes around. Drizzle everything with the extra-virgin olive oil, sprinkle the pomegranate molasses or balsamic vinegar over the tomatoes and season the whole dish with salt and pepper. Roughly tear the basil and mint leaves over the top, keeping small ones whole as they look beautiful.

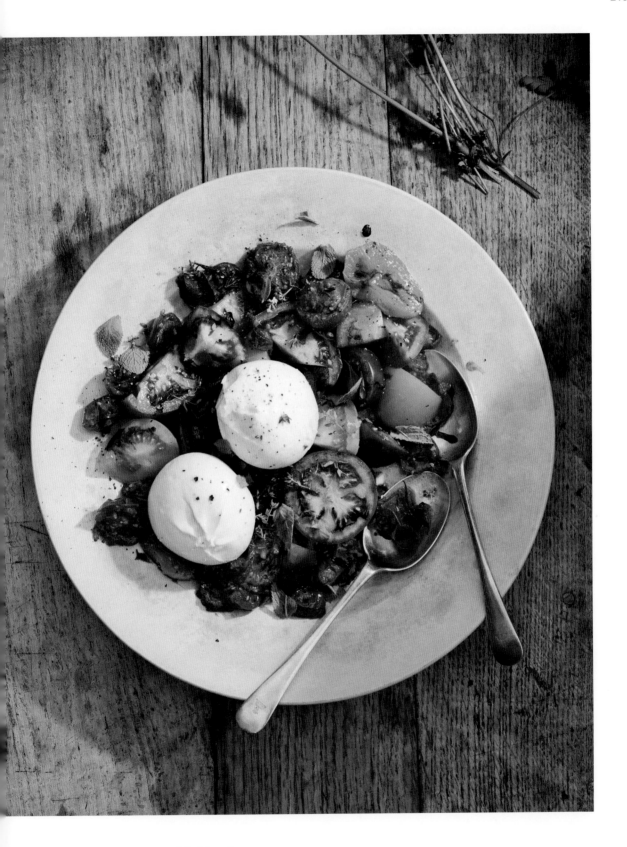

stress-free sharing with friends

veggie party platter

Who doesn't love a party platter?! I like to make a couple of elements and then use shop-bought bits too – take a look at the platter overleaf for an example. You could prepare some to keep in the fridge so you have 'building block' snacks ready for when you have a snack attack.

sweet potato rounds and roasted chickpeas with whipped feta and harissa honey

feeds 4–6 as a party side ——— 30 minutes

2 tbsp olive oil or melted ghee
400g tin of chickpeas, drained
  and rinsed
2 medium sweet potatoes,
  skin on, sliced into rounds
2 tsp *(rose)* harissa paste
Sea salt and black pepper

whipped feta and harissa honey
200g feta
200g Greek-style yoghurt
1 garlic clove, finely chopped
2 tsp dried oregano
1 tsp *(rose)* harissa paste
1 tbsp runny honey

to serve
Cucumber, chopped
Red chicory leaves and Little
  Gem leaves

Preheat the oven to fan 220°C/gas mark 9, then divide the olive oil between two large roasting trays and place in the oven to heat up.

Meanwhile, dry the rinsed chickpeas in a clean tea towel so that they don't spit in the hot oil as they roast.

Place the sweet potato in one of the trays, rub both sides of each sweet potato in the hot oil and lay flat, spaced apart, then sprinkle over a little salt and pepper. Scatter the chickpeas in the second roasting tray and toss in the hot oil with the harissa paste and a generous pinch of salt and some pepper.

Pop both the sweet potato and the chickpeas in the oven to roast for 25 minutes. Halfway through the cooking time, remove both trays. Flip over the sweet potato rounds to cook on the other side and carefully shake the tray of chickpeas. Swap both trays round (so that the one that was on the top shelf moves to the middle shelf, and vice versa) and place back in the oven to continue cooking.

For a smoother finish, place the feta, yoghurt, garlic and half the oregano in a food processor with 1 tablespoon of water, then season with salt and pepper and blitz. Alternatively, for a more rustic texture, mash the feta in a bowl before mixing with the other ingredients.

Transfer to a serving bowl, mix the harissa paste and honey together and drizzle over the whipped feta before sprinkling with the rest of the oregano. Serve with the roasted chickpeas and sweet potato on the side, as well as the cucumber and salad leaves. The roasted chickpeas add great texture on top of the whipped feta and also on hummus and other dips.

sticky spiced nuts and seeds

feeds 4 as a party side ——— 10 minutes

2 tbsp ghee, butter or oil
2 large handfuls of mixed nuts
  *(such as cashews, almonds
  and pistachios)*
1 large handful of mixed seeds
  (such as pumpkin or nigella seeds)
2 tsp curry powder or garam
  masala
A pinch of cayenne pepper
2 sprigs of rosemary or thyme
  or 1 tsp dried herbs
2 tbsp maple syrup or runny
  honey
Sea salt and black pepper

Heat up the ghee in a large frying pan while you mix all the other ingredients except the maple syrup/honey in a bowl and season with salt and pepper.

On a low–medium heat, let the nuts fry nice and gently for 4–5 minutes, taking care not to burn – they will smell incredible! You can spread these over a large baking tray and pop in the oven at fan 180°C/gas mark 6, but I find it easier to keep an eye on them on the hob as they can burn easily.

Stir every now and then to make sure the nuts and seeds are coated in the spices and herbs and getting toasted, then drizzle in the maple syrup or honey, stir and cook for another 45 seconds before tipping everything back into the bowl.

Leave to cool for at least 10 minutes before eating – they will crisp up as they cool. Add another sprinkling of salt, if you like, to serve.

Store any leftovers in a clean screw-top jar with tight-fitting lid and use for sprinkling on soups or salads.

sun-dried tomato tapenade

feeds 4–6 as a party side ——— 5 minutes

150g pitted black olives
4 large sun-dried tomatoes
1 garlic clove
1 tbsp capers
1 ½ tbsp balsamic vinegar
A pinch of chilli flakes
150ml extra-virgin olive oil
1 handful of fresh parsley or
  basil, roughly chopped
Sea salt and pepper, to taste

Roughly chop the olives, sun-dried tomatoes and garlic, then combine everything except the olive oil and herbs in a food processor. Blitz, slowly drizzling in the olive oil as you go, until you get to a nice chunky consistency.

Taste for seasoning, there are lots of salty flavours so you may not need to add any extra sea salt. Stir in the herbs, reserving a little to serve. Transfer to a small bowl and top with the remaining herbs.

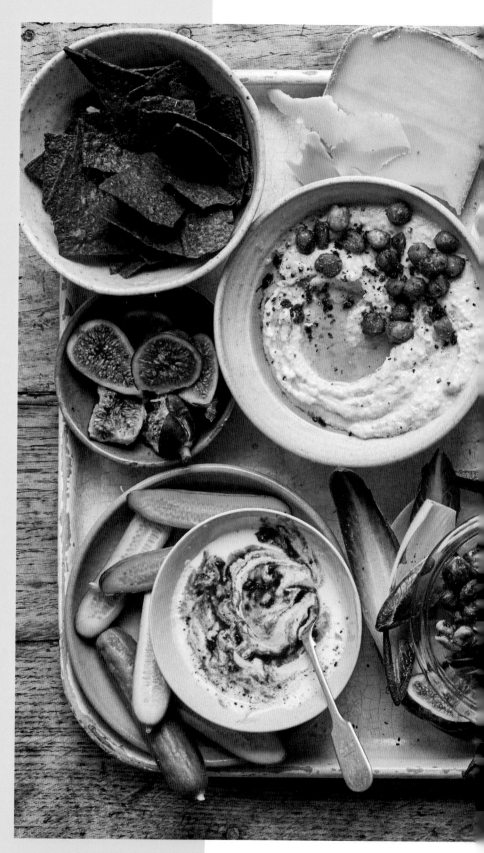

Clockwise from bottom left:
Whipped Feta and Harissa
Honey (page 214), Hummus
(page 63) Sweet Potato Rounds
(page 214), Roasted Chickpeas
(page 214), Farinata (page 218),
Sticky Spiced Nuts and
Seeds (page 215)

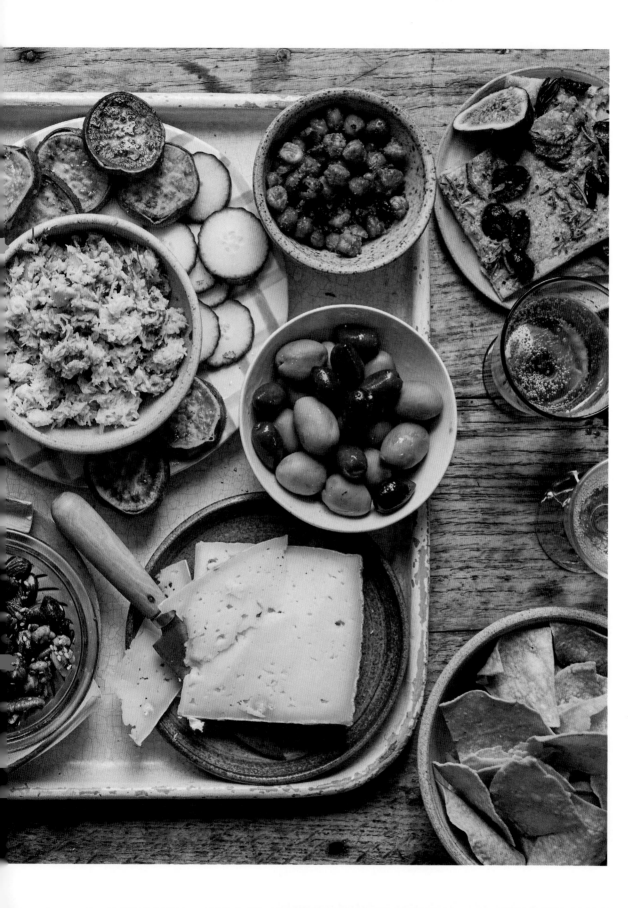

farinata

makes 8 slices ——— 40 minutes *(hands-on time 10 minutes)*

150g chickpea *(gram)* flour
5 tbsp olive oil
1 ¼ tsp sea salt, plus extra for
  sprinkling on top
Good pinch of black pepper
1 red onion, finely sliced
20 pitted black olives, halved
6 sprigs of rosemary

A must make. Here chickpea batter is baked into a thin, crispy pancake that is perfect for dipping into **Hummus** (page 63) or to have alongside the beautiful **Hearty Spiced Veg Stew** on page 42 and other soups.

Place the flour in a big jug or mixing bowl and slowly pour in 300ml of water, whisking as you go.

Preheat the oven to its highest temperature. Take your largest baking tin, approx 30cm × 22cm (if you don't have one this large, use two smaller tins approx 22cm × 18cm). Grease the base and sides with 1 tablespoon of the olive oil and place in the oven to heat up.

Whisk the remaining 4 tablespoons of olive oil into the flour mix, along with the 1¼ teaspoons of salt and lots of black pepper.

Remove the hot tin(s) from the oven, pour in the batter and top evenly with the onion, olives and the rosemary sprigs. Bake for 30 minutes until deeply golden and crisp on top. (Check after 20 minutes and turn down the temperature to fan 200°C/gas mark 7 if it's getting too dark.) Let the farinata cool in the tin(s) for 15 minutes (if you can wait that long!) before slicing each one into quarters and serving with an extra sprinkling of salt on top.

variation

Swap half the olives
for 6 anchovies.

feel good

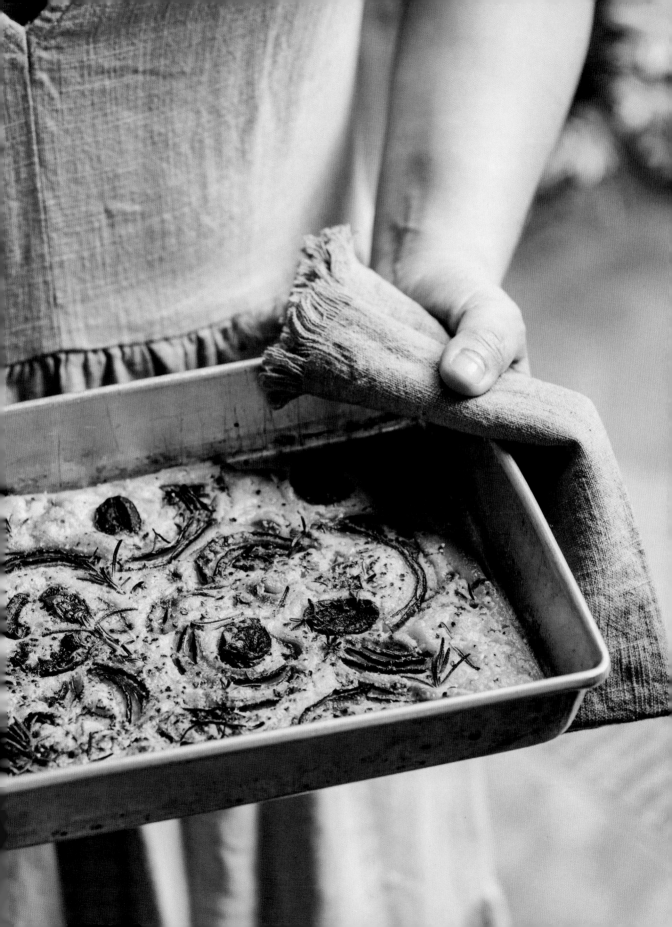

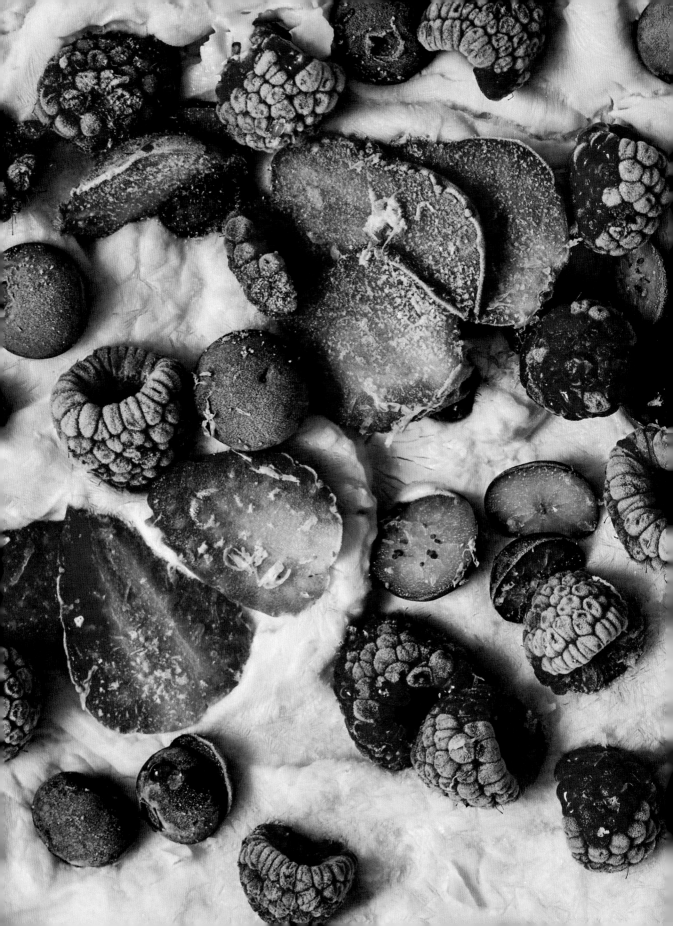

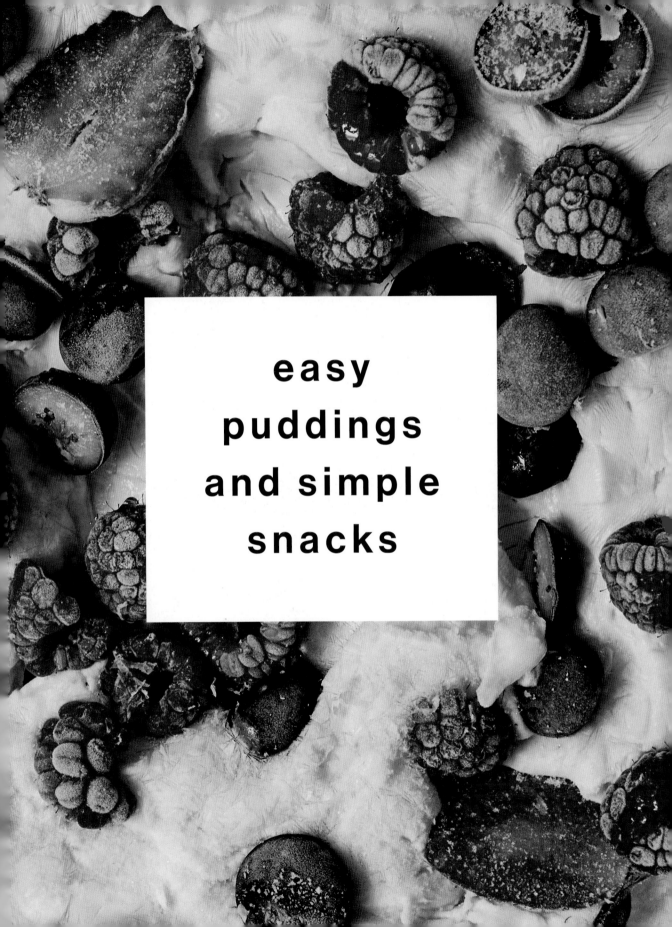

easy
puddings
and simple
snacks

/ these recipes are deliberately simple /

From bakes to no-bakes, and hot-day sweets to cosy-up treats, there's something here for everyone. As I don't have a hugely sweet tooth, I mostly use fresh or frozen fruit to add sweetness, or small amounts of maple syrup, honey or coconut sugar. The eggs used in a couple of the baked dishes can easily be swapped for a plant-based alternative (see page 245 for how to make a 'flax egg').

I love using oats in baking because they're easy to get hold of and affordable, and can even be ground into flour. You'll see that I also use ground almonds because of the flavour and, as a result, all of these recipes are naturally gluten-free. They're also deliberately simple and most of them come together in one bowl, so no need for fancy equipment and extra washing-up. All the recipes can be prepped ahead and most can be frozen – win-win!

For a portable snack, keep a little stash of the **Fruity Oat Bites** on page 234 (I love popping a few in my pocket for a long walk) or the **No-bake Chewy Nutty Bars** (page 227) that you refrigerate rather than bake and that last for ages stored in the fridge.

For a stress-free dinner party, make the **Three-Ingredient Chocolate Pots** (page 230); you can prep them in advance and they happen to be vegan too, so everyone can enjoy them. Peckish working from home? Have a chocolate-coated date stuffed with almond butter and a tiny sprinkling of sea salt (for that unbeatable sweet–salty combo). So simple and hits the spot every time. If you can get hold of pistachio or hazelnut butter, then wow, all the better!

PS: As a Fairtrade ambassador, I always recommend looking out for the Fairtrade logo when you're shopping. From chocolate to sugar, vanilla extract to cinnamon, bananas, tea and much more, Fairtrade products are widely available, in both big and small shops and from big and small brands alike, and buying them is a great way to give support and help guarantee fair prices for farmers globally.

In other chapters, look out for:

- **15-minute Frying-pan Granola** (page 35)
- **Blueberry Ricotta Pancakes** (page 32)
- **Sticky Spiced Nuts and Seeds** (page 215)

chocolate-coated stuffed dates

makes 12 ——————— 20 minutes + chilling for 1 hour

80g dark *(50%–70%)* chocolate, broken into squares

2 tsp coconut oil

12 big Medjool dates *(see introduction)*

2–3 tbsp almond butter or other nut butter or tahini *(stirred well in the jar first)*

Sea salt

for rolling

10g peanuts or flaked almonds

10g desiccated coconut

10g pistachios *(look out for the raw bright green ones)*, chopped

Keep extras stored in the fridge in an airtight container, they will keep for a week. Avoid dried, firm dates; they need to be soft and squidgy for this recipe – I like Medjool. Freeze-dried raspberries or crushed dried rose petals make a delicious and beautiful option for rolling the stuffed dates. See my tip for a quick version of this recipe.

First, toast the peanuts or flaked almonds for 3–4 minutes in a small frying pan on a medium heat until just going golden. Toss them in the pan as they cook, then remove from the heat and set aside to cool.

Meanwhile, set up a bain-marie: place a heatproof bowl on top of a small saucepan of simmering water (making sure the base of the bowl does not touch the water), add the chocolate and coconut oil and leave to melt. Take off the heat once fully melted and stir to combine.

Roughly chop the toasted peanuts (if using) and sprinkle on a small plate, along with the desiccated coconut and the pistachios. Line a tray or large plate with baking parchment.

Remove the pits from the dates and use a teaspoon to stuff each of the dates with about ½ teaspoon of the nut butter or tahini (it gets a little fiddly here). Squidge together the sides of each date to close it up as best as you can, then spear the date with a fork and dunk it a few times into the melted chocolate. Dunk fully or just half.

Place on the lined tray or plate, then sprinkle and press over the coconut or nuts. Sprinkle with a tiny pinch of salt and repeat with the other dates. You should end up with three batches of four chocolate-coated dates, each batch rolled in one of the three different nut options, but mix and match as you like.

Place the plate or tray in the fridge to chill for about 1 hour until set. Bring them out about 15 minutes before eating for the best taste and texture.

tip

If you're in a rush, simply stuff the pitted dates with nut butter and pop in a square of dark chocolate, then bite straight into it.

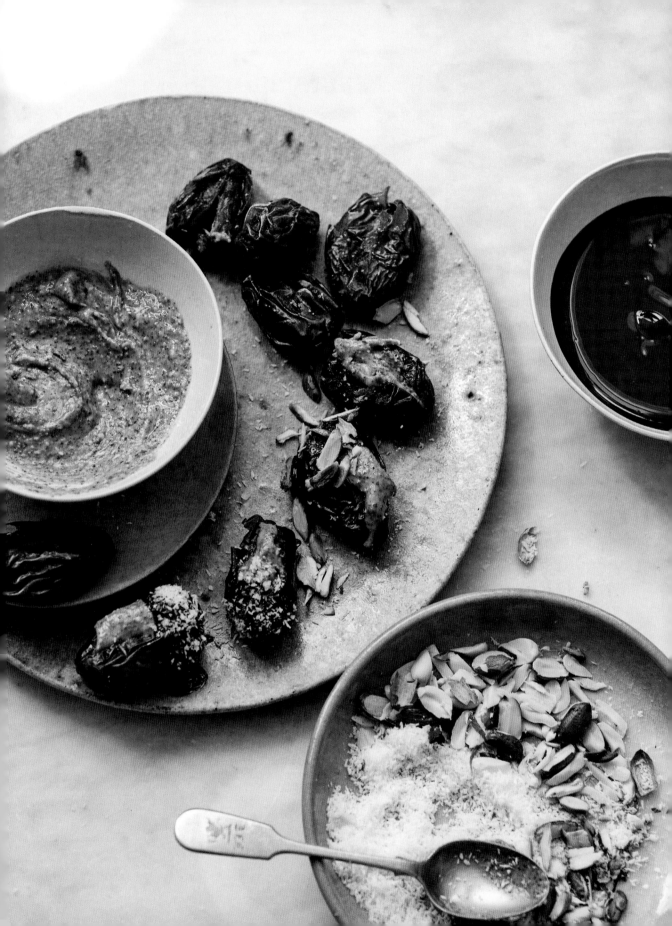

no-bake chewy nutty bars

makes 16 bites ——————— 20 minutes + chilling for 3 hours

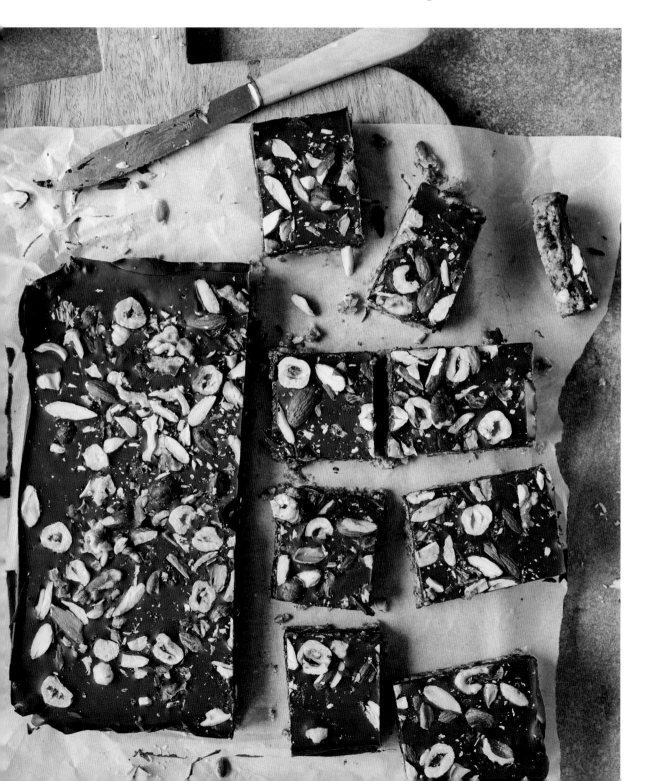

150g mixed whole walnuts,
hazelnuts and almonds,
roughly chopped
200g dark *(50%–70%)*
chocolate, broken into squares
5 tbsp coconut oil
240g pitted Medjool dates
200g ground almonds
2 tsp vanilla extract
½ tsp sea salt
80g roughly chopped pistachios
(or pumpkin seeds), for topping

Any nuts and seeds work in these delicious bars. I've made them with just hazelnuts before for a lovely praline flavour. You might like to swap the vanilla extract for a dash of peppermint or orange extract, or add a bit of rum and a few raisins or some toasted coconut flakes. You could also top with dried rose petals for a beautiful gift. Or add a little pinch each of ground cinnamon, cloves and nutmeg and ground or candied ginger with dried cranberries for a festive touch at Christmas? These are best served straight from the fridge for the ultimate chewiness!

Start by toasting the whole nuts (not the pistachios) for 5 minutes in a large frying pan on a medium heat until fragrant and just going golden. Toss them in the pan as they cook and watch them like a hawk after 3 minutes!

Next, set up a bain-marie: place a heatproof bowl on top of a small saucepan of simmering water (making sure the base of the bowl does not touch the water), add the chocolate and 2 tablespoons of the coconut oil and leave to melt until smooth, stirring from time to time. Once melted, set aside to cool slightly.

Add the dates, ground almonds, vanilla, remaining coconut oil and salt to a food processor and pulse until combined and dough-like.

Add 50g of the toasted nuts (roughly a third, it doesn't need to be exact) and pulse again briefly until roughly ground but still with some slightly larger bits, and then turn off the machine and stir in the pistachios or pumpkin seeds to make a nice balance of squidgy dough and crunchy nuts and seeds.

Line a rectangular tin about 25cm × 20cm and 4cm deep – and transfer the mixture from the food processor to the tin. Press down really well with your hands to make a nice and flat, compact layer.

To finish, pour the glossy melted chocolate mix on top to create a thick layer, using a spatula to get every last lovely drop out of the bowl. Scatter with the rest of the toasted nuts and the chopped pistachios and pop in the fridge for 3 hours, until the chocolate layer is nice and hard, which makes it easy to slice and lovely to chew. Bring the tin out of the fridge for 10 minutes before slicing into 16 squares. Keep stored in the fridge. These will last for a few weeks in a sealed container.

tip

The bars will be easier to slice if you run some hot water over a sharp knife before using.

easy puddings and simple snacks

oaty choc-chunk cookies

makes 14 cookies ——— 25 minutes *(hands-on time 10 minutes)*

1 medium ripe banana, peeled *(about 110g)*

1 egg

4 tbsp maple syrup

1 tsp vanilla extract

120g smooth nut butter *(such as almond butter, stirred well in the jar first)*

80g dark *(50%–70%)* chocolate *(or a mix of raisins and chocolate)*, chopped into 5mm cubes

120g rolled oats *(not quick-cook oats)*

80g ground almonds

1 tsp baking powder

⅛ tsp sea salt, plus extra for sprinkling *(optional)*

Use a soft, very ripe banana as this will give natural sweetness to these chewy oaty cookies. I like to keep them chunky so they are nice and soft. Make sure you space them out and use two baking trays if you need to. Any cookies not eaten straight away can be kept in a biscuit tin for 3 days.

———————————————————————

Preheat the oven to fan 190°C/gas mark 6½ and line a large baking tray with baking parchment.

In a large mixing bowl, mash the banana with a fork, then push to one side of the bowl, crack in the egg and whisk with the fork. Add the maple syrup, vanilla and nut butter and mix everything together.

Place the chocolate chunks in a second bowl, saving a few tablespoons for pressing on top of the cookies, then add all the other ingredients and mix together.

Add the contents of the second bowl to the first bowl and stir all the ingredients together. Using two spoons, place dollops of the mixture on the prepared baking tray, spaced apart, to create 14 equal-sized cookies. (I like them nice and rustic, rather than too neatly shaped.) Press some of the reserved chocolate chunks into each cookie.

Bake for 13–15 minutes until golden at the edges and firm-ish to the touch (they are lovely if they are still a bit soft in the middle). I recommend sprinkling a tiny extra bit of salt on top of each cookie before leaving to cool on the tray for 10 minutes (where they'll continue cooking) and then transferring to a wire rack to sit for another 10 minutes before eating.

tip

Freeze cooled cookies, then defrost and bake before eating.

variation

Instead of using just dark chocolate chunks, try a mix of raisins and chocolate.

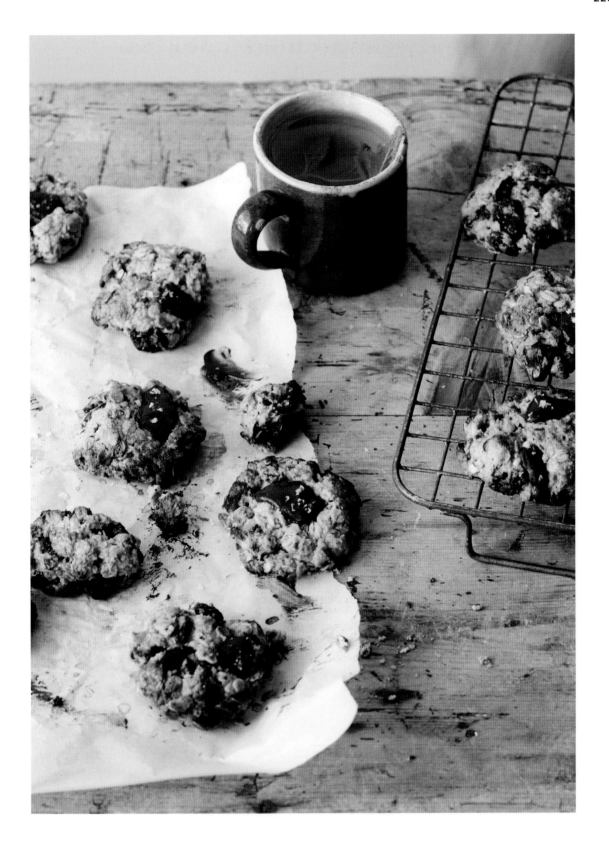

easy puddings and simple snacks

three-ingredient chocolate pots

feeds 6 ———— 20 minutes + 4 hours chilling

180g Medjool dates *(about 10 large dates)*
250ml nut milk
160g dark *(50%–70%)* chocolate
A little pinch of sea salt, plus extra to serve *(optional)*

optional toppings
Dollop of *(plant-based)* cream
Chopped toasted hazelnuts or pecans
Pitted cherries or fresh pomegranate seeds
Raspberries or strawberries
Crushed biscuits *(such as ginger nut or digestive)*

These are so simple and delicious, plus they're plant-based! If you want to make them in advance, they'll keep for 3 days in the fridge. I love them made with just the three ingredients – hazelnut milk works particularly well – but if you want to go to town, try adding extra toppings – whatever you have in your cupboard! These are quite rich, so they happily feed six. You'll need 6 ramekins or glasses/jars – tea cups would look lovely; just avoid delicate glasses that might crack under the hot mix.

Roughly tear the dates, discarding the pits, and soak in just-boiled water for 10 minutes. Even though Medjool dates are soft anyway, this helps soften them further, which is good for any blenders that might need a helping hand.

Heat up the nut milk in a saucepan, being careful not to boil, and remove from the heat once it's heated through.

Meanwhile, finely slice about 2 tablespoons of the chocolate to create some chocolate 'shavings' and set aside for garnishing.

Chop the rest of the chocolate and add to a blender or food processor, then pour over the hot nut milk. Drain the soaked dates and add them with the salt, then carefully blend until smooth.

Divide the mixture between 6 ramekins or glasses (see introduction) and chill in the fridge for 4 hours until set. Cover them if you're keeping them there any longer, so they don't pick up 'fridge' smells. Scatter over the chocolate shavings, plus a tiny extra sprinkle of sea salt, if you like, or add any of the other toppings to serve.

variation

For a Christmassy chocolate-orange flavour, add ½ teaspoon orange extract to the blender and top the finished pots with a little grated orange zest. Add a festive flourish of a tiny pinch of nutmeg or cloves.

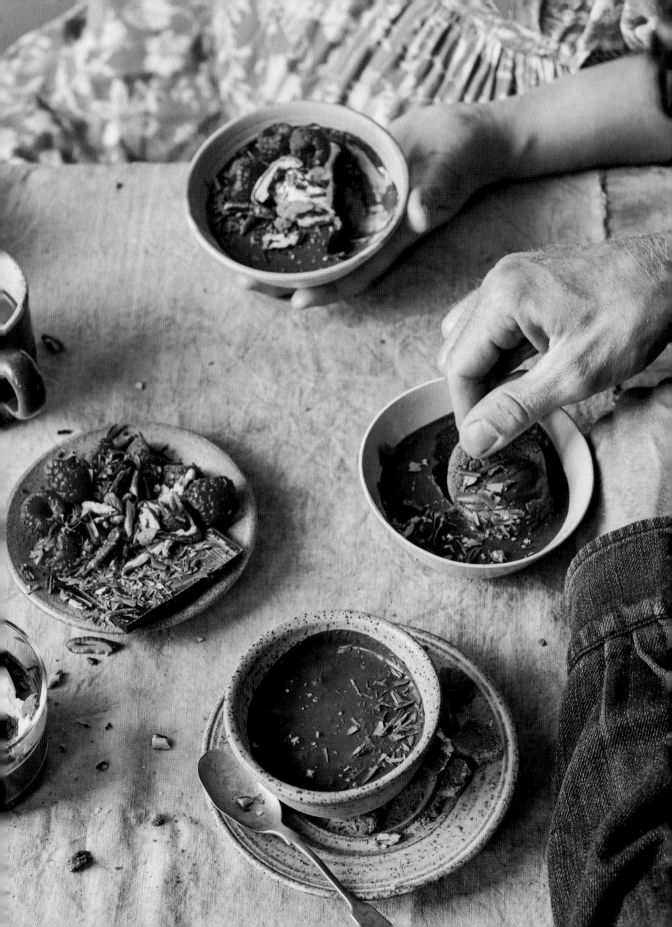

banana and blueberry bake

makes 8 hearty slices ———— 1 hour 10 minutes
(hands-on time 15 minutes)

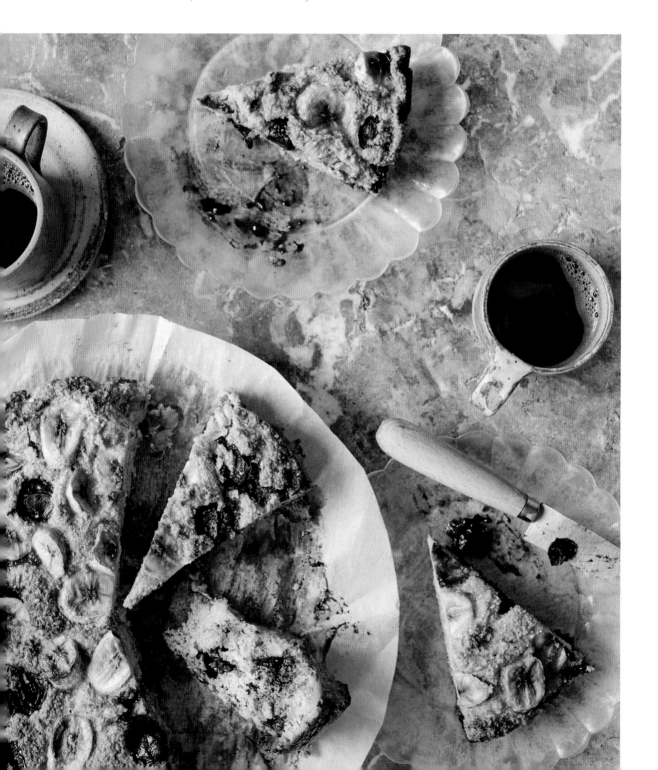

30g unsalted butter or coconut oil, plus extra for greasing

3 very ripe medium bananas, peeled *(350g)*

A tiny pinch of sea salt

3 tbsp maple syrup

1 tsp ground cinnamon

1 tsp vanilla extract

3 eggs

1 tsp bicarbonate of soda

Juice of ½ lemon and 1 tsp grated zest

200g ground almonds

3 tbsp ground flaxseed

100g blueberries *(fresh or frozen)*

I've combined two favourites here – banana bread and blueberry muffins. I bake this all year round with fresh berries in the summer and frozen berries when they're out of season. This would also be glorious with raspberries or, come autumn, blackberries picked from a hedgerow. I have made this with cherries and chocolate chunks too – oh my! The ripe bananas add natural sweetness, enhanced by a little maple syrup, which make it good for breakfast too, but if you want it sweeter, add another tablespoon of maple syrup.

Preheat the oven to fan 170°C/gas mark 5. Meanwhile, melt the butter in a small saucepan, then remove from the heat and allow to cool slightly.

In a big bowl, mash two and a half of the bananas to a pulp with a fork, saving the remaining half banana to decorate the top of the cake.

Add the melted butter, sea salt, maple syrup, cinnamon, vanilla, eggs, bicarbonate of soda and lemon juice and zest. Mix together well with a whisk.

Add the ground almonds and flaxseeds and mix well. Stir in a third of the blueberries (no need to defrost them if frozen).

Grease a 23cm round cake tin really well with butter and line with baking parchment, then pour in the batter, smooth the top and decorate with the remaining half banana, sliced into 8 thin 'coins', and the rest of the blueberries.

Bake for 40 minutes, then turn down the heat to fan 160°C/gas mark 4 and bake for a final 15–20 minutes until a skewer inserted into the middle of the cake comes out clean. (If using fresh blueberries, it will probably only need 15 minutes of the final baking time, if using frozen it will probably need 20.) Allow to cool in the tin before removing from the tin and slicing to serve. Store any leftovers in an airtight tin.

variation

If you want to bake muffins, grease a 12-hole muffin tin or line with paper cases. Divide the batter between the moulds and bake for 40–45 minutes.

fruity oat bites

makes 22 bites ——— 30 minutes *(hands-on time 10 minutes)*

3 tbsp unsalted butter
200g rolled oats
2 small very ripe bananas *(200g)*
3 tbsp smooth nut butter *(such as almond or cashew, stirred well in the jar first)*
4 tbsp mixed dried fruit *(such as raisins and chopped apricots)*
2 tsp ground cinnamon
A tiny pinch of sea salt, plus extra for sprinkling

These are lovely for a mid-afternoon snack with a cup of tea. Choose coconut oil instead of butter to make it plant-based; I love both versions equally. The sweetness all comes from the dried and fresh fruit, so make sure the bananas are very ripe. Use your favourite nut butter for these: I do find, though, that peanut butter tends to be make these little bites a bit drier so I prefer almond or cashew.

Preheat the oven to fan 190°C/gas mark 6½ and line a large baking tray with baking parchment.

Melt the butter in a medium saucepan, then add the oats and cook on a medium heat for 4–5 minutes, stirring a few times, to achieve that delicious golden, toasted flavour.

Meanwhile, mash the bananas very well with a fork in a medium bowl.

Add the nut butter to the oats and stir until mixed, then remove from the heat. Add the mashed banana and all the remaining ingredients and stir until combined. If you have time, wait 10 minutes for the mix to cool down a little, as it makes it easier to form the fruit bites.

Take about 2 teaspoons of the mix and roll it into a ball in your hands, pushing down any dried fruit into the mix, as they might burn if left poking out on top. Repeat with the rest of the mixture until you have 22 small bites, and place, spaced apart, on the baking tray.

Bake for 10 minutes until golden-edged and, once out of the oven, leave for 10 minutes on the tray before transferring to a wire rack to cool for another 15 minutes. Enjoy straight away or store somewhere cool, in a biscuit tin or airtight container, for up to 5 days.

variation

Replace the ground cinnamon with a pinch of ground ginger or chai spice mix.

feel good

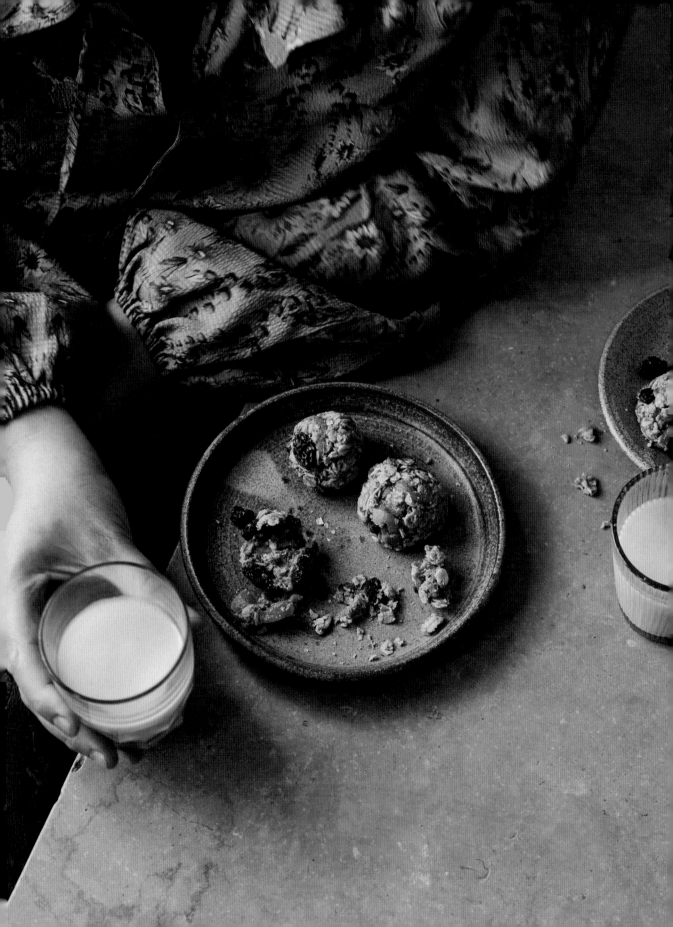

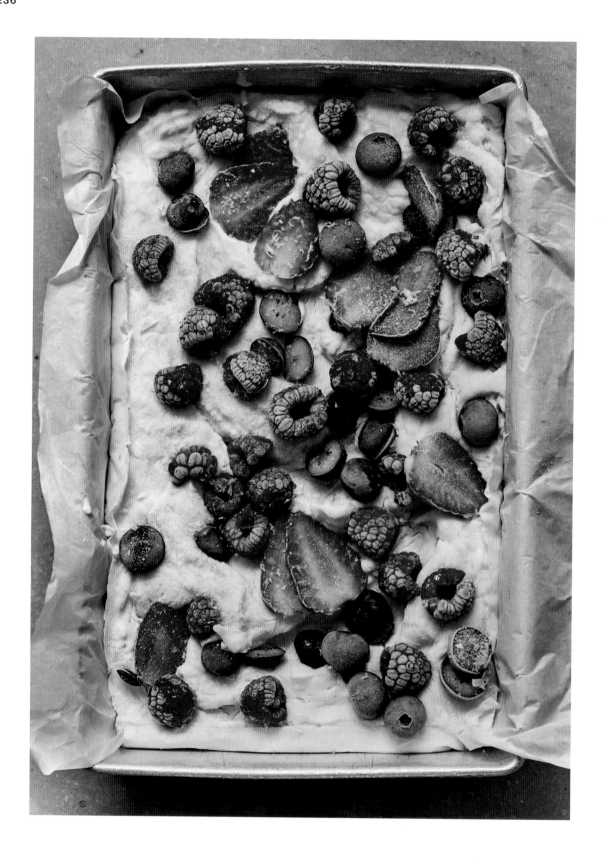

frozen yoghurt bark ~ two ways

makes 1 tray ——————— 10 minutes *(hands-on time)* + freezing for 3–4 hours

yoghurt bark

250ml thick yoghurt
  (Greek-style or coconut)
3 tbsp runny honey or maple
  syrup
1 tsp vanilla extract *(optional)*
1 tsp lime or lemon juice
A tiny pinch of sea salt

mixed berry version

125g mixed berries *(strawberries
  and other larger berries sliced)*
1 tbsp nuts *(such as flaked
  almonds or chopped pistachios
  – optional)*
2 tbsp pomegranate seeds
  (optional)

tropical fruit version

150g sliced mixed tropical fruits
  *(such as mango, papaya, kiwi
  and banana)*
1 ½ tbsp desiccated coconut
A little grated lime or lemon zest

As you may have experienced when making ice cream, if you eat something frozen, you don't taste the sugar as much, so I really recommend adding the sweetener, vanilla extract, citrus juice and salt to bring out the sweetness. Trust me: this will take it to the next level! You can use frozen or fresh berries here. Frozen are more likely to bleed, but that's fine, it will just look different to my one, pictured.

Line a medium baking tray (one that can fit in your freezer) with baking parchment. You'll want it to be at least 1.5cm deep.

Mix the yoghurt with the all the other ingredients for the basic yoghurt bark (see tip) and spread out on the lined tray to about 1cm thick. (The mixture can be thicker, depending on the size of your baking tray, but I prefer biting into thinner pieces of the frozen yoghurt bark.)

Scatter your choice of fruit over the yoghurt and then scatter over any nuts, seeds or desiccated coconut and citrus zest, if using.

Pop into the freezer for 3–4 hours until the yoghurt is set, then break it roughly into shards or slice into thin rectangles and enjoy straight away. Keep any leftover pieces in a sealed container in the freezer.

tip

I usually stir the other ingredients straight into the yoghurt pot, to save a bowl, but you can mix everything together in a bowl, if you prefer, or blend it with some of the fruit for colour.

flavour-saver fruity ice cubes

5 minutes + freezing for 2–3 hours

flavour-saver options

Fresh mint or basil leaves

Leaves from sprigs of rosemary or thyme

Cucumber slices

Chopped apple or pear

Strawberries, raspberries or blueberries

Small wedges of lemon, lime, orange or grapefruit

Thin slices of ginger

to serve

Juice of ½ lemon

Sparkling water

Splash of gin or vodka per glass *(optional)*

Perfect for adding refreshing flavour to sparkling water and for using up any odds and ends you may have in your fridge – fresh herbs, a solitary apple or pear in your fruit bowl or the last few berries in a punnet. Make these ice cubes 2–3 hours before you serve your drinks.

Fill up an ice-cube tray with any of the flavour-saver options, top up with cold water and pop into the freezer for 2–3 hours until set.

Pour the ice cubes into a large jug, add the lemon juice then top up with sparkling water, add a splash of gin or vodka to each glass, if you like, and serve. Cheers!

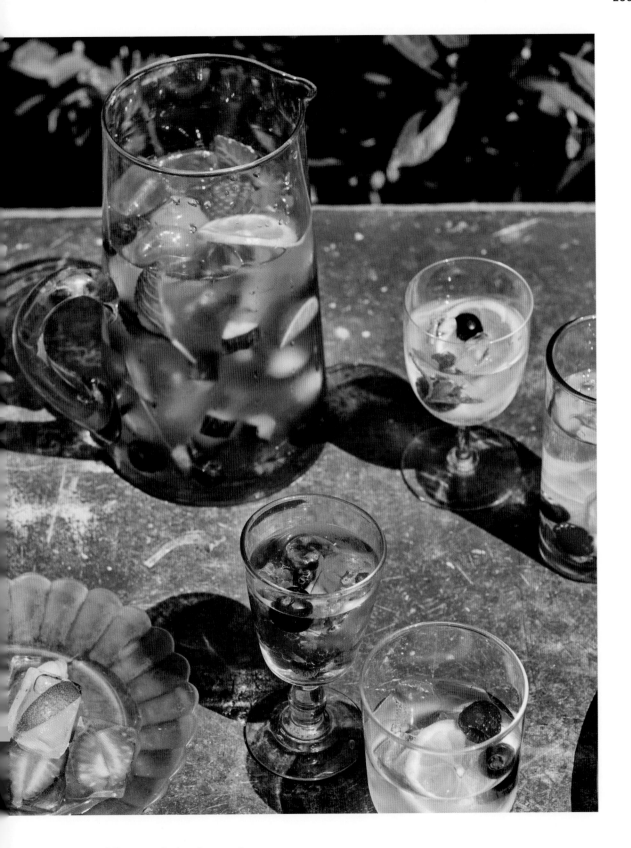

easy puddings and simple snacks

recipe round-ups

One-pot wonders and traybakes
- Baked Eggs with Harissa Chickpeas and Zhoug, page 23
- Baked Eggs with Sage Mushrooms and Whipped Goat's Cheese, page 24
- One-pan Pesto Chickpeas and Broccoli, page 123
- Cauliflower, Cannellini and Cherry Tomato Traybake, page 142
- Halloumi Veg Traybake with Chilli-Honey Drizzle, page 144
- One-pot Sweet Potato and Spinach-Lentil Bake, page 149
- Pesto-Mozzarella Baked Aubergines, page 165
- Spiced Feta-Meatball Traybake, page 174
- Spiced Chickpea and Fish Traybake with Garlic Yoghurt, page 182
- One-pan Oregano Chicken and Chickpeas, pages 192–4

Half-hour heroes
- Zingy Vietnamese-style Noodles with Fried Sesame Tofu, page 131
- Cosy Coconut Lentils with Kachumber, page 64
- Scrambled Spiced Tofu, page 18
- Broccoli Coconut Curry Soup, page 53
- Quick Broccoli, Mushroom and Sweet Potato Soup, page 57
- Baked Feta and Ras el Hanout Broccoli Salad, page 79
- Crab and Courgette Spaghetti, page 112
- Sesame Noodle Salad with Quick-pickled Cucumber, page 125
- Creamy Mushroom and Spinach Pasta, page 128
- Fried Halloumi and Chickpea Rainbow Salad, page 150
- Shiitake Mushroom Adobo, page 154
- Mum's Filipino Chicken, page 179
- Sesame Fish with Tricolour Quinoa, page 191
- Black Bean and Sweet Potato Wraps with Chipotle Mayo, page 203

Store-cupboard-friendly recipes to lean on
- 15-minute Frying-pan Granola, page 35
- Store-cupboard Soup Five Ways, pages 44–5
- Speedy Chickpea and Frozen Kale Coconut Curry, page 60
- Roasted White Beans with Caesar-style Tahini Dressing, page 76
- Quick Leeky Beans, page 94
- Store-cupboard Sardine Puttanesca with Tagliatelle, page 126

Best for batch cooking and freezer filling
- Hearty Spiced Veg Stew, page 42
- Hummus Bowls with Bean Bites, page 63
- Any Bean, Any Lentil Chilli, page 66
- Veg-packed Mac 'n' Cheese , pages 114–16
- Spaghetti and Veg Balls in Tomato Sauce, pages 120–2
- Beans and Greens Golden Broth, page 54
- Half-and-Half Cottage Pie with Cheesy Parsnip Mash, pages 176–8

Pick-me-ups – snacks to have on standby
- 15-minute Frying-pan Granola, page 35
- Smoked Mackerel Pâté, page 82
- Sticky Spiced Nuts and Seeds, page 215
- Oaty Choc-Chunk Cookies, page 228
- No-bake Chewy Nutty Bars, page 227
- Fruity Oat Bites, page 234
- Frozen Yoghurt Bark Two Ways, page 237

Prep ahead for busy weeks
- Breakfast Muffins with Banana, Carrot and Seeds, page 36
- Baked Oats Three Ways, pages 28–9
- Sweetcorn-Carrot Fritters, page 146
- Lunchbox 'Chuna' Two Ways, page 186
- Lunchbox Orzo Pasta Salad, page 189
- Sweet Potato Salad with Peanut-Lime Sauce, pages 102–3
- Sweet Potato Fishcakes, pages 195–7
- Three-Ingredient Chocolate Pots, page 230

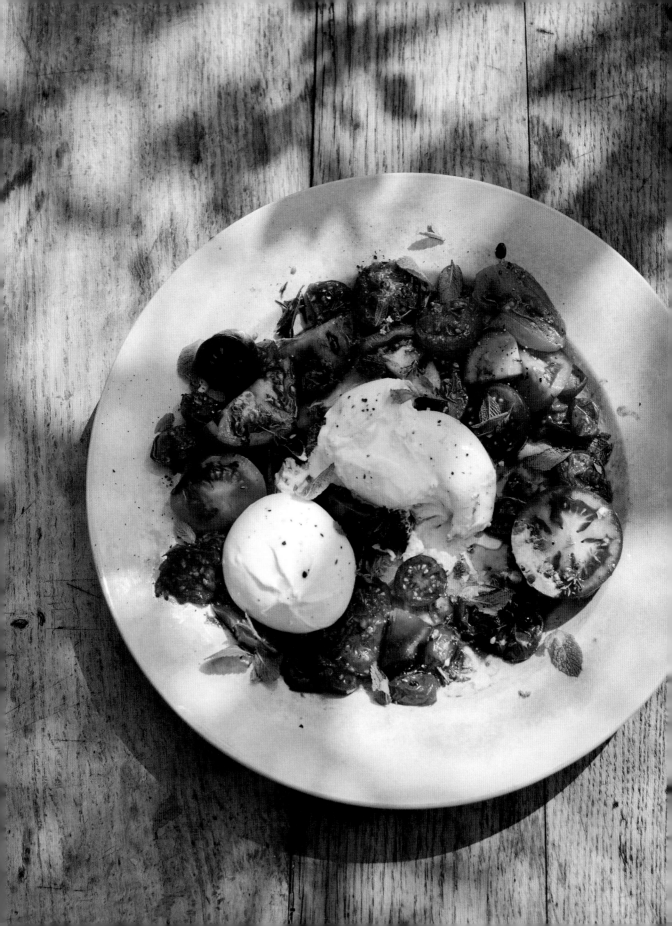

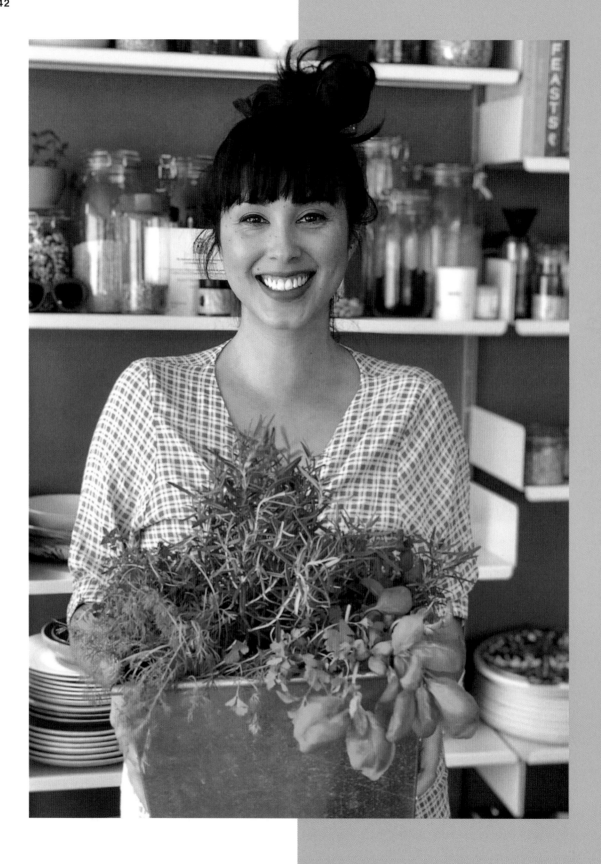

easy ways to pump
up the flavour

- Add some umami oomph to dressings, sauces, soups, stews, noodle broths and gravies with a few teaspoons of tamari, soy or Worcestershire sauce, or you could even add 1 teaspoon of fish sauce or miso or some chopped anchovies to a bolognese sauce.

- Go for very large roasting trays and large frying pans to ensure that vegetables and other ingredients like chickpeas and beans are well spaced so that they roast and fry without steaming, which helps concentrate the flavour.

- Dry ingredients well after washing, or after draining and rinsing, in order to concentrate the flavour and prevent the ingredients from spitting when added to hot oil. Be sure to dry salad well to allow the dressing to coat the leaves properly, otherwise it will slide straight off.

- Where you can, cook your quinoa, rice or buckwheat in veg stock rather than water and add a bay leaf or a pinch of dried mixed herbs when cooking beans or lentils.

- Some of my favourite flavour boosters to always keep on hand include (rose) harissa paste, curry paste and homemade chicken stock. (Freeze stock in ice-cube trays and pop them out as needed.)

- My go-to homemade spice mixes and dressings include **shawarma** (page 162), **Red Miso Sauce** (page 72) and **Peanut-Lime Sauce** (page 102). You could make up a triple batch of each of these and keep the shawarma spice mix in a sealed jar for a few months and the other two in the fridge for a few weeks.

- Sometimes a simple squeeze of lemon or lime juice or a little finely grated zest on top of a salad, dip or soup can brighten up a dish and bring out the flavours. A touch of vinegar will give a sharp lift too.

- Herbs, dried or fresh, really pack a punch. Don't forget the flavour in the fresh herb stems too. Check out the **Chimichurri Drizzle** (page 90), **Pesto** (page 123) and **Coriander-Lime Drizzle** (page 203).

- Make homemade pickles like the **Quick-pickled Veg** or two types of **pickled red onions** (page 246) for adding extra flavour to dishes.

- Keep a jar of delicious fermented kimchi or sauerkraut to top noodle salads and stews.

- Save your Parmesan rinds and pop them into soups, risottos, broths and tomato sauces for pasta to add extra flavour during cooking.

- I always recommend using sea salt, seasoning as you cook, tasting as you go and seeing if you need a little sprinkling at the end to finish.

- Sweet baked dishes almost always benefit from a tiny sprinkling of sea salt.

- Freshly ground black pepper makes such a difference.

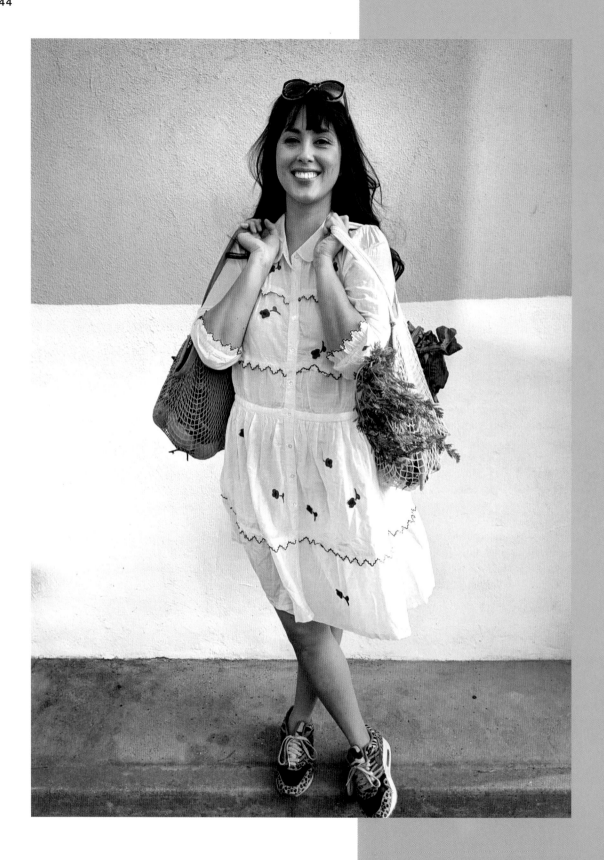

tips and swaps for vegan friends

- 1–2 tablespoons of nutritional yeast add a fantastic depth of flavour to dishes such as the **Lemony Spinach and Feta Quinoa** (page 134) and cheesy pasta sauces.

- Look out for vegan/plant-based Worcestershire sauce and fish sauce.

- Use seaweed sprinkles (ground seaweed) or seaweed salt in broths, soups and stir-fries.

- Finely chopped and fried mushrooms make a great alternative to minced meat, as do brown lentils.

- To add creaminess to dressings, curries and dips, use tahini, nut butter or coconut cream, milk or yoghurt.

- Swap honey for maple syrup or coconut sugar.

- For briny saltiness straight from the store cupboard, add chopped olives, capers or jalapeños from a jar.

- Make **homemade pickles** such as the ones on page 246.

- Keep a jar of delicious fermented kimchi or sauerkraut to top noodle salads and stews.

- Replace 1 egg with 1 'flax egg'. Add 1 tablespoon of ground flaxseed to a small bowl with 3 tablespoons of water, stir together well and leave for 5 minutes. If you can only find whole flaxseed, either grind to a fine powder using a pestle and mortar before mixing with the water, or blitz the mixture in a very powerful blender or the small bowl of a food processor.

- For more ways to add depth of flavour, see the previous page.

go-to sauces and pickles

These are my favourite additions to so many recipes! If you'd like to make them ahead of time, they will keep for about a week in the fridge.

spicy mayo

makes 1 small bowl —— 5 minutes

2 tbsp mayonnaise
1 tsp toasted sesame oil
1–2 tsp chilli sauce or chilli oil *(to taste)*
2 tsp tamari or soy sauce

Mix all the ingredients in a small bowl. Season with salt to taste.

quick-pickled onion

makes 1 bowl —— 5 minutes
+ pickling for 5 minutes

1 big red onion, halved and very finely sliced
Juice of 2 limes *(or 1 big lemon)* and a little grated zest, or 3 tbsp apple cider vinegar
¾ tsp sea salt

Place the red onion in a bowl with the lime (or lemon) juice and zest (or the vinegar) and salt. Scrunch and massage the onion in the lime juice for 30 seconds, then leave to bathe in the salty citrus juice for 5 minutes, where it willl go bright pink and delicious.

spicy lime-pickled red onion

makes 1 small bowl —— 5 minutes
+ pickling for 20 minutes

Juice of 2 limes
1 tsp runny honey or maple syrup
1 small red onion, finely sliced
1 garlic clove, finely chopped
½ tsp ground cumin
1 fresh jalapeño, deseeded and finely chopped, or a pinch of chilli flakes
A pinch of sea salt

Mix everything together in a small bowl and leave to 'quickly pickle' for 20 minutes.

quick-pickled veg

makes 1 bowl —— 5 minutes
+ pickling for 10 minutes

½ small red onion, finely sliced
Juice of 1 lime
2 tsp maple syrup
A generous pinch of sea salt
⅓ cucumber, finely sliced
1 large carrot, scrubbed and finely sliced
1 handful of finely sliced radishes or cabbage

Place the onion in a medium bowl with the lime juice, maple syrup and salt and leave to 'pickle' for about 10 minutes before mixing with the remaining ingredients to serve.

freestyle fruit-bowl chutney

makes 1 jar ——— 35 minutes *(hands-on time 20 minutes)*

5 medium eating apples
(unpeeled) or 2 large
  ripe mangos *(about 900g)*
2 tbsp ghee or coconut oil
1 tsp sea salt
½ tsp black pepper
½ tsp ground turmeric
½ tsp ground cinnamon
6 tbsp maple syrup
120ml apple cider vinegar

spice paste
3 garlic cloves, peeled
1½ tbsp roughly chopped
  fresh ginger
1 tbsp coriander seeds or 2 tsp
  ground coriander
1–2 fresh chillies, deseeded if
  you prefer and chopped, or
  a pinch of chilli flakes *(to taste)*

For when your fruit bowl is groaning! I love this with apple or mango, as here, or a mixture. It would be great with tomatoes too. Delicious with **curries** (pages 48 and 60) or the **Shawarma-inspired Cauliflower and Sweet Potato Bowls** (page 162), or on **Sweetcorn-Carrot Fritters** (page 146). Stir a little into dressings or yoghurt for dipping and drizzling.

First make the spice paste. Place the garlic, ginger, chillies and coriander seeds, if using, in the small bowl of a food processor and blitz to a fragrant paste, or pound everything together with a pestle and mortar. If you're not using coriander seeds, then just finely chop everything and mix together with the ready-ground coriander.

Chop the apples into 1cm pieces or, if using mango, cut up the peeled mango flesh into slightly bigger pieces.

Heat up a small saucepan and melt the ghee, then add the spice paste, salt, pepper, turmeric and cinnamon and gently fry on a low heat for 2–3 minutes, stirring regularly.

Stir in the fruit, then add the maple syrup and vinegar and simmer, uncovered, for 15–20 minutes, stirring a few times, until thick and just like a chutney. Remove from the heat and taste for seasoning: it should be a delicious, lip-smacking balance of sweet and sour. Allow to cool – it will thicken further as it cools – and then pop into a clean screw-top jar. It will keep for about a week in the fridge.

cook's notes

- All recipes were tested using a fan oven. Oven temperatures may vary so keep an eye out for visual cues.

- Some recipes have 'hands-on time' stated, when the time it takes is a lot longer than the time you will spend in the kitchen so you can let the hob and the oven do the hard work.

- Spring onions are whole (using both the green and white parts) unless otherwise stated. No waste!

- Unwaxed lemons/limes can be used for zesting, or add the peels to your drinks.

- Fresh herbs are whole (with stalks included) unless otherwise stated.

- Ginger only needs to be peeled if it is not organic.

- Save veg scraps (squash peel, herb stalks, onion skin) to make veg stock or compost if you can.

- When I have time, I try to soak and cook dried beans and chickpeas from scratch as it's cheaper and more sustainable. The recipes all use tinned cooked beans and chickpeas as most of us find them the most convenient.

- When using veg or drained cooked beans and chickpeas in roasting recipes, dry them well in a clean towel and use a wide roasting pan to prevent steaming from overcrowding.

- Plant-based options can always be used for dairy items (milk, yoghurt, etc.). See page 245 for vegan tips and swaps.

- Dairy items (milk, ricotta, yoghurt, cream cheese) are whole/full-fat. Coconut milk is also full-fat.

- Butter is salted unless stated otherwise.

- Eggs are always medium and free range, ideally organic, and kept at room temperature.

- Source the best quality animal products (eggs, dairy, meat) that you can. For responsibly sourced fish, ask your fishmonger for advice on what's available. If your local shop doesn't stock organic, you'll find many farmers online delivering direct to your door.

- Sea salt is always flaked.

- If you haven't got all the ingredients, especially when it comes to vegetables, don't worry, you'll spot variations or feel very welcome to be flexible with the recipe, swap carrot for squash or spinach for kale and be inspired by the seasons.

- Cook once, eat twice! Most of the recipes are suitable for freezing. Why not double up and freeze the leftovers for a rainy day or just roll over the extra portions into dinner another day this week?

- Look out for the refill aisle in your local shop or supermarket. It's great to see more and more refill shops opening all over the UK. I like to cut back on plastic packaging by doing a monthly top up of my dried goods in these shops – they are great for stocking up on basic items like pasta and rice plus you can buy small amounts of ingredients that you're less familiar with to try them out.

thank you to . . .

Lizzie Mayson and Kitty Coles for bringing the recipes to life with your gorgeous photography. I feel very lucky to work with you and your brilliant shoot team – Ollie Grove and styling assistants Clare Cole, Joanna Jackson, Flossy McAslan and Valeria Russo. Thanks for putting in such hard work and for all the packing-up-leftovers-to-take-home compliments. What a confidence boost.

For great cheer and calmness in the chaos of book-making, thanks to Sarah Malcolm (also for shooting the front cover and the other pictures of me) and to Florence Blair for support in styling, proofing, triple-recipe-testing and more.

Natasha Crawley, Jenny Fyans, Evangelina Hemsley, Ruth Sanders, Shelley Martin-Light, Fiona Hemming and Eva Ramirez... all your testing made the recipes even better.

Team Found – especially Alice Russell, KJ Sullivan and Daisy Janes. For giving me the support, time and space to write this book and be me.

My book family at Ebury Press, our fifth cookbook together – as always to the wonderful Lizzy Gray for championing me, and to my editors Emily Brickell and Celia Palazzo, as well as Stephenie Reynolds, The Happy Foodie team and Lucy Harrison. Nikki Dupin at Studio Nic&Lou for designing. And of course Sarah Bennie PR for all her energy and kindness over the last 10 years.

Friends who have inspired me and encouraged me to spend much more time on my mental health and find the confidence to talk about it – Nadiya Hussain, Dr Rupy Aujla, Fearne Cotton, June Sarpong, Donna Lancaster, Bryony Gordon, the Mental Health Mates community, Kimberley Wilson, Brigid Moss and Emma Cannon, and my guests from The Feelgood Sessions.

Booksellers around the world, for stocking my books in your wonderful bookshops.

Henry Relph, Mum and Nelly for looking after me while I looked after the book.

Last but not least, a gigantic thank you to you for reading and cooking from *Feel Good*. It has been a joy to make. I very much hope you enjoy it with your loved ones. Thank you for your support and happy cooking!

You'll see I am inspired by my travels and influenced by cuisines all over the world, but I am not an expert in all of them. The recipes in this book are my take on the dishes I have loved. Some of the many chefs who have inspired me in my cooking are: Imad Alarnab, of Imad's Syrian Kitchen, Melek Erdal, Lara Lee, Sabrina Ghayour, Rachel Ama, Romy Gill, Ravinder Bhogal, Asma Khan, Amy and Emily Chung, Craig and Shaun McAnuff, Food With Mae and Uyen Luu. If you're on Instagram, you'll see me cooking with lots of these wonderful chefs in my video series of Cook Together Cook Alongs, follow me there: @melissa.hemsley

index

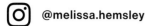 @melissa.hemsley

 @melissahemsley

 @melissahemsleycooks

melissahemsley.com

1

Ebury Press an imprint of Ebury Publishing,
20 Vauxhall Bridge Road,
London SW1V 2SA

Ebury Press is part of the Penguin Random House group of companies
whose addresses can be found at global.penguinrandomhouse.com

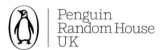
Penguin
Random House
UK

First published by Ebury Press in 2022
www.penguin.co.uk

A CIP catalogue record for this book is available from the British Library

Design: Nikki Dupin at Studio Nic&Lou
Cover design: Luke Bird
Photography: Lizzie Mayson, except pages 2, 8, 242 and 244
Cover photography and photos on pages 2, 8, 242 and 244: Sarah Malcolm
Food and prop styling: Kitty Coles

ISBN 978-1-52910-981-8

Colour origination by Altaimage Ltd, London
Printed and bound in Germany by Firmengruppe APPL, aprinta druck, Wemding

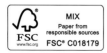

Penguin Random House is committed to a sustainable future for our business, our readers and our planet.
This book is made from Forest Stewardship Council® certified paper.

Bestselling author Melissa Hemsley is a cook, writer and champion of sustainable home cooking that supports the way you feel. She creates simple, veg-packed and delicious recipes that comfort and delight any night of the week.

She began her food career as a private chef for international actors and bands, including Take That, and has written and co-written four bestselling books, published internationally: *The Art of Eating Well*; *Good + Simple*; *Eat Happy* and *Eat Green*. *Feel Good* is her fifth book.

Melissa is a proud supporter of food waste charity The Felix Project, and volunteers with them regularly to rescue surplus food and to cook for children and the vulnerable. She is an ambassador for Mental Health Mates, the Fairtrade Foundation and Women Supporting Women (The Prince's Trust), among others.

She hosts three of her own event series: The Sustainability Sessions, Cook Together Cook Alongs and The FeelGood Sessions, where she chats to leading experts, well-known faces and fellow chefs about everything from their mental wellbeing to planet-friendly kitchen tips.

Melissa regularly appears on cookery and news shows, often speaking on behalf of the charity and community projects she works with.

She lives with her boyfriend and dog in East London, where she cooks, writes, tries to grow veg and feeds a steady stream of hungry friends, happily squeezed around her kitchen table.

Find out more about Melissa and watch her 'Kitchen How-To' videos on her Instagram @melissa.hemsley